# First Aid
## for Babies and Children
### *fast*

## LONDON, NEW YORK, MUNICH, MELBOURNE, DELHI

**Consultant Editor** Jemima Dunne
**Senior Editor** Janet Mohun
**Editorial Assistant** Lili Bryant
**Designers** Jacqui Swan, Fiona Macdonald
**Jacket Designer** Mark Cavanagh
**Managing Editor** Camilla Hallinan
**Managing Art Editor** Michelle Baxter
**Production Editors** Rebekah Parsons-King, Francesca Wardell
**Production Controller** Mary Slater
**Publisher** Sarah Larter
**Art Director** Philip Ormerod
**Associate Publishing Director** Liz Wheeler
**Publishing Director** Jonathan Metcalf

First published in Great Britain as First Aid for Children Fast in 1994;
revised in 1999, 2002, and 2006
This fifth edition published 2012 by Dorling Kindersley Limited,
80 Strand, London WC2R 0RL
A Penguin Random House Company

6 8 10 9 7 5

005–188427–Oct/2012

A CIP catalogue record for this book is available from the British Library
ISBN 978-1-4093-7912-6

Printed and bound in China by C&C Offset Printing Co., Ltd

Discover more at
**www.dk.com**

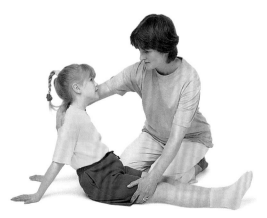

# Foreword

Children are naturally adventurous and suffering minor injuries is all part of growing up, as are childhood illnesses. Fortunately serious injuries and illnesses rarely happen, but it is important that a child receives the best possible first aid if they do. Good care can not only preserve life, but it can also speed up the recovery process. This revised edition of *First Aid for Babies and Children Fast* contains the latest guidelines for life-saving procedures as well as guidance on how to deal with those minor injuries and illnesses.

This book is published in association with the British Red Cross, an organisation that helps people in crisis worldwide. In the UK, the British Red Cross provides first aid education for millions of people every year, building not only personal skills but community resilience, helping people to cope with all types of first aid emergencies.

I hope the contents of this book will not only provide you with the knowledge and skills to look after a child who has suffered a minor injury or illness, but will also help you to feel more confident and willing to take action if a more serious emergency occurs.

Log onto *childrenfirstaid.redcross.org.uk* for free first aid advice online. Watch videos, animations and download additional first aid information to help you learn valuable skills.

Dr Vivien J Armstrong MBBS FRCA DRCOG PGCE (FE)
Chief Medical Adviser to the British Red Cross

# Contents

# Introduction

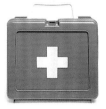

This book has been compiled primarily for parents but also for others – grandparents, teachers, childminders, playgroup leaders, and babysitters – who may regularly, or even occasionally, find themselves in charge of infants and children. The content has been set out in a clear and logical way and the information presented largely in pictorial form using simple words and captions to make it very easy to follow and to understand. The first aid advice given can be used to treat any age child up to puberty and follows the most up-to-date clinical guidance at the time of publication.

Emergencies are, by their very nature, unexpected events and can be extremely frightening and stressful for anyone caring for a child. *First Aid for Babies and Children Fast* will help you to learn various practical skills that will help you to cope with a range of first aid emergencies and everyday accidents, building your confidence and ensuring that you respond in the best way possible. The calmer you are the more effective your help will be, and by listening and talking to the child you will be able to make the best decision for both you and him or her, greatly improving the outcome.

The British Red Cross regularly runs a wide range of first aid courses specifically designed for the care of babies and children. You can find out more by visiting www.redcross.org.uk or calling 0844 412 2808. There are also online learning resources available where you can access first aid information at anytime of day, visit *childrenfirstaid.redcross.org.uk* to watch videos, test your skills, and download information.

# How to use this book

This book covers first aid treatment for everything from minor cuts and grazes to treating an unconscious child. For every condition a series of photographs shows you

Key signs and symptoms help you to recognise the conditions

Annotations highlight essential action

Clear photographs illustrate every step of treatment

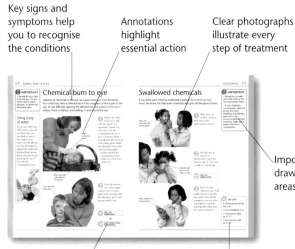

Symbols highlight the action necessary for medical help

Cross-references direct you to pages with information about associated injuries

exactly what to do in an emergency. Key pieces of information are indicated on the photographs and supplementary advice can be found alongside in the step-by-step text.

The injuries are organised by type, in coloured sections such as Wounds and Bleeding and Bites and Stings. However, in an emergency, the thumbnail index on the back cover will direct you straight to the relevant page. There are also sections, such as Action in an Emergency, Bandages and Dressings, and Home Safety, that contain information for general reference.

Important boxes draw attention to areas of concern

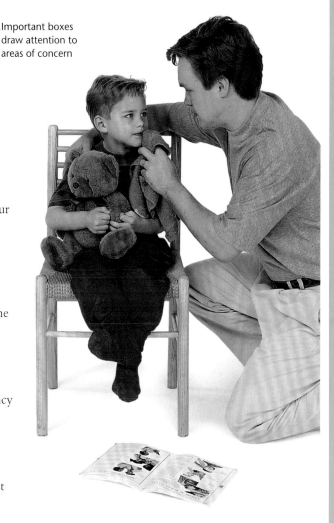

## GUIDE TO THE SYMBOLS

The following symbols and instructions appear if your child needs further medical attention:

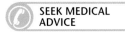

**SEEK MEDICAL ADVICE**

Depending on your area, call your doctor's surgery, nurse practitioner, duty paramedic, NHS direct, or the local NHS walk-in centre for advice.

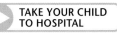

**TAKE YOUR CHILD TO HOSPITAL**

Take your child to the nearest accident and emergency department if you have help and transport.

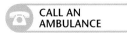

**CALL AN AMBULANCE**

Your child needs urgent medical attention and is best transported by ambulance to hospital.

# Action in an emergency

In any emergency, particularly one involving children, it is important to keep calm and act logically. Remember four steps:

 **Assess the situation**

- What happened?
- How did it happen?
- Is there more than one injured child?
- Is there any continuing danger?
- Is there anyone who can help?
- Do I need an ambulance?

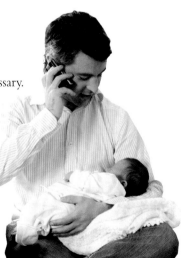

## Think of safety

- Do not risk injuring yourself – you cannot help if you become a casualty.
- Remove any source of danger from your child.
- Move your child only if you must for her safety and do so very carefully.

## Treat serious injuries first

In children, there are two conditions that immediately threaten life:
- Inability to breathe (see UNCONSCIOUSNESS *p.14*).
- Serious bleeding – this is usually obvious and can be brought under control (*see p.44*).

> **! IMPORTANT**
> - **If** more than one child is injured go quickly to the quiet one – she may be unconscious.

## Get help

Shout for help early and ask others to:
- Make the area safe.
- Seek medical advice or call an ambulance.
- Help with first aid.
- Move a child to safety, if necessary.

## Telephoning for help

When you call the emergency services, ask for an ambulance. The following information will be helpful:
- Your telephone number.
- The location of the incident.
- The type of incident.
- The number, sex, and ages of the casualties.
- Details of injuries.
- Information about hazards such as gas, power lines, or fog.

# Fire

Write down an escape plan for your home and make sure everyone knows what to do.
- How would you get out of each room?
- How do you help babies and young children?
- Where will you meet when you've escaped?

## Action for a chip pan fire

- Turn off stove or hob, then cover pan with lid, wet tea towel, or fire blanket – leave this on for half an hour – NEVER throw water over the flames.
- If fire is not under control, get out of the house, closing doors behind you, and call the fire brigade.

## Escaping from a fire

 Feel the door. If the door is cool, leave the room.

**OR**

 If the door is hot, don't open it. Go to the window.

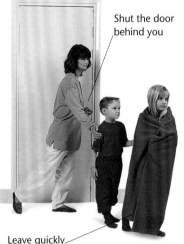

Shut the door behind you

Leave quickly
DO NOT GO BACK

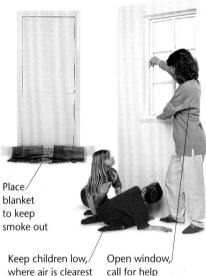

Place blanket to keep smoke out

Keep children low, where air is clearest

Open window, call for help

### ⚠ IMPORTANT

- **Carry** babies and toddlers.
- **Don't** ask children to do anything other than look after themselves.
- **Close** all doors behind you.
- **Meet** outside your house.
- **Never** go back inside.
- **Phone** for help from elsewhere.

**If you have to escape through a window:**

- **If** you have to break the glass, put a blanket over the frame before you escape.
- **Slide** your child out, hang onto him, then ask him to drop down.
- **Slide** out yourself, hang from the ledge, then drop.

## Clothing on fire

**If clothing is on fire:**
**Stop** your child moving as movement will fan the flames.
**Drop** him to the floor and wrap him in a coat or blanket to help smother the flames.
**Roll** him on the ground.

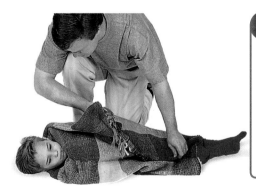

### ⚠ IMPORTANT

- **Do not** let your child run about in a panic; rapid movement will fan the flames.
- If water is available, lay him down, burning side uppermost, and douse him with water or a non-flammable liquid.

### ! IMPORTANT

● **Never** touch your child's skin. Pull at his clothes as a last resort.

● **If** your child is unconscious, open his airway and check breathing. If breathing, place in the recovery position; if not breathing, begin rescue breaths and chest compressions.

## High-voltage current

Contact with electricity from power lines and overhead cables is usually fatal. Severe burns result and the child may be thrown some distance from the point of contact. NEVER approach the child unless you know for sure that the power has been cut off.

### ≫  see also

● Electrical burns, p.60

● Unconscious baby, pp.17–21

● Unconscious child, pp.22–29

# Electrical injury

Children are at risk of electric shock if they play with electrical sockets or flexes. Electrical current causes muscle spasms that prevent a child letting go of an electric cable and may cause burns both where it enters and leaves the child's body. In extreme cases, the current may also cause breathing and heart to stop.

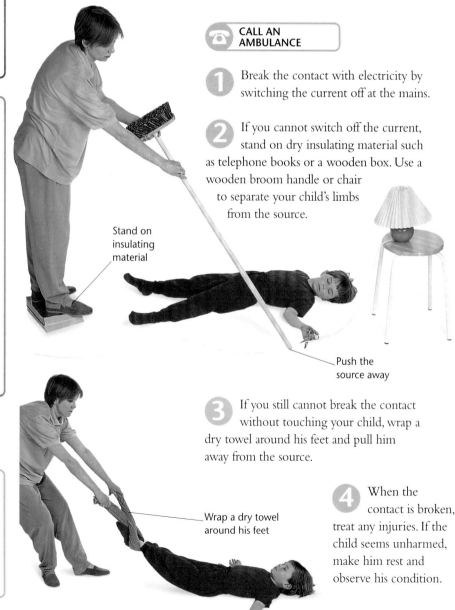

Stand on insulating material

Push the source away

Wrap a dry towel around his feet

### ☎ CALL AN AMBULANCE

**1** Break the contact with electricity by switching the current off at the mains.

**2** If you cannot switch off the current, stand on dry insulating material such as telephone books or a wooden box. Use a wooden broom handle or chair to separate your child's limbs from the source.

**3** If you still cannot break the contact without touching your child, wrap a dry towel around his feet and pull him away from the source.

**4** When the contact is broken, treat any injuries. If the child seems unharmed, make him rest and observe his condition.

# Drowning

Babies and young children can drown quickly if they slip into a pool or pond or are left unattended in a bath. Even 2.5cm (1in) of water is enough to cover a baby's nose and mouth if she falls forwards.

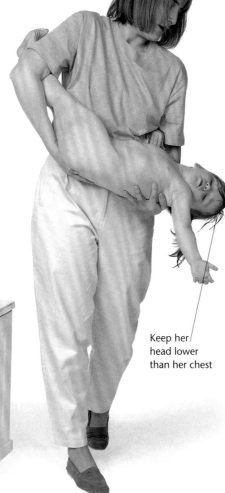

Keep her head lower than her chest

**1** Lift your child out of the water. Carry her with her head lower than her chest to reduce the risk of inhaling water.

**2** Remove any wet clothing and cover her with a dry towel or blanket.

**3** If your child is unconscious, open the airway and check breathing. If breathing, place her in the recovery position; if she is not breathing, begin rescue breaths and chest compressions.

> **CALL AN AMBULANCE**

---

## ! IMPORTANT

● **If** you need to give rescue breaths you may need to blow into the child's mouth more firmly and more slowly than usual to get the chest to rise. Water and the effects of cold can increase resistance to rescue breathing.

● **Always** seek medical advice even if she appears to have recovered. She may have inhaled some water, which can cause lung damage.

## Rescue in open water

A child may get into difficulty in open water especially if it is turbulent or very cold. Rescue her quickly. Try to reach her from the shore or bank with your hand, or with a stick. Get her dry and warm as quickly as possible.

## ≫ see also

● Hypothermia, *p.90*

● Unconscious baby, *pp.17–21*

● Unconscious child, *pp.22–29*

# Unconsciousness

A baby or child needs to inhale oxygen into his or her lungs. This oxygen passes into the bloodstream and is pumped around the body by the heart. If a baby or child is unconscious, the airway to the lungs may be blocked so oxygen can't enter the body. Lack of oxygen slows down the heartbeat until it stops (cardiac arrest) and no oxygen will reach the brain.

## What you can do

If a child is unconscious, you must open the airway. Then, if necessary, breathe into the lungs (rescue breathing). If circulation stops, oxygenated blood cannot travel to the brain so you need to drive the blood to the brain with chest compressions. This combination is known as cardiopulmonary resuscitation (CPR). A machine called an AED (automated external defibrillator) can be used to restore a normal heartbeat in a child over the age of one (*see p.23*).

Always make sure it is safe to approach the baby or child; you can't help if you become a casualty too. When you are certain you are safe, assess whether he or she is conscious, then follow the ABC of resuscitation: A for airway, B for Breathing and C for Compressions.

## Chain of survival

An unconscious baby or child's chances of survival are greater if:
- You call for expert help;
- CPR is given as soon as possible;
- A defibrillator is used early;
- Advanced care by paramedics and hospital is received as soon as possible.

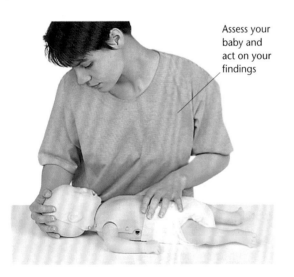

Assess your baby and act on your findings

Assess your child and act on your findings

Tap his shoulder

# A is for airway

You need to open the air passage, or airway. Place one hand on the forehead and gently tilt the head back to bring the tongue away from the back of the throat. If you suspect a neck injury, use the jaw thrust method to open the airway (*see p. 70*).

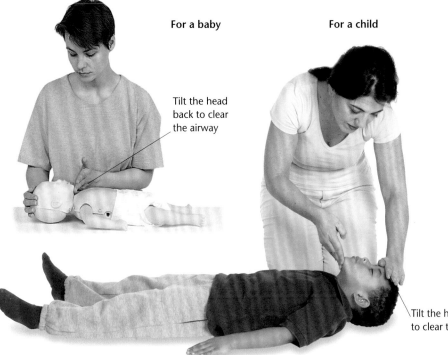

**For a baby**

Tilt the head back to clear the airway

**For a child**

Tilt the head back to clear the airway

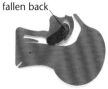

## Airway

If child is on his back the tongue falls back and blocks the airway.

Tongue fallen back

**Blocked airway – head not tilted**

Tongue forward

**Unblocked airway – head tilted**

# B is for breathing

If your child is not breathing after the airway has been opened, take a breath and blow steadily into the lungs to get oxygen into the child's blood.

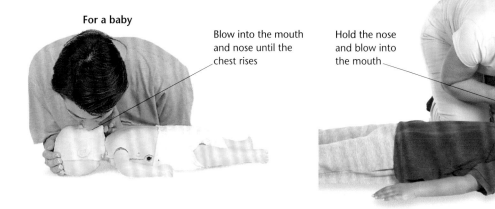

**For a baby**

Blow into the mouth and nose until the chest rises

**For a child**

Hold the nose and blow into the mouth

# C is for compressions

If your child's heart has stopped, giving chest compressions will drive blood containing oxygen around the body. This will be more effective if combined with rescue breathing. The combination of techniques is known as cardiopulmonary resuscitation (CPR).

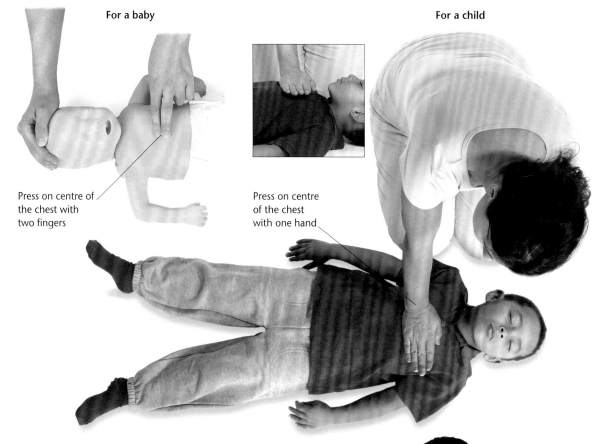

**For a baby**

**For a child**

Press on centre of the chest with two fingers

Press on centre of the chest with one hand

## When to call an ambulance

If there is somebody else present to help, always ask him or her to call an ambulance as soon as you realise that your child is not breathing. If you are on your own, give rescue breaths (*see* rescue breathing: baby *p. 18*; child *p. 24*) and chest compressions (*see* CPR: baby *p. 20*; child *p. 26*), for 1 minute before pausing to call an ambulance.

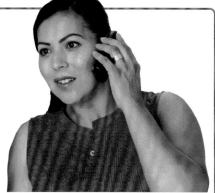

# Unconscious baby

Assess your baby before calling for help. If you are alone and the baby is not breathing, begin rescue breaths and chest compressions.

## 1 Check for response

- Call her name, or tap her foot gently. Never shake a baby.
- If there is no response, continue to step 2.
- If there is a reponse,

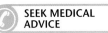
**SEEK MEDICAL ADVICE**

Call her name

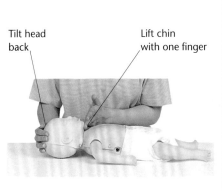

## 2 Open baby's airway

- Put one hand on the baby's forehead and gently tilt her head.
- Place one finger of your other hand on the tip of her chin and lift it.

Tilt head back

Lift chin with one finger

### ! IMPORTANT
- **Do not** press the soft part of the neck under the chin as it can block the airway.

## 3 Check breathing for up to 10 seconds

- Look, listen, and feel for breathing. Look along her chest for movement, listen for sounds of breathing, and feel for breaths against your cheek. Send helper to:

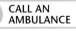
**CALL AN AMBULANCE**

Listen for breaths

Look for chest movements

Feel for breath on your cheek

- If she is breathing, cradle her in your arms with head tilted down and wait for help.
- If she not breathing give five initial rescue breaths – GO TO PAGE 18.

### Resuscitation summary

Unconscious baby

⬇

Airway open

⬇

No breathing

⬇

Send helper to

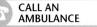
**CALL AN AMBULANCE**

⬇

Give five initial rescue breaths

⬇

Begin CPR (30 chest compressions alternating with 2 rescue breaths)

⬇

Repeat for 1 minute

⬇

If not already done,

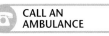
**CALL AN AMBULANCE**

⬇

Continue CPR until help arrives

### ! IMPORTANT
- **If** you are unable or unwilling to give rescue breaths you can give chest compressions only.

### Resuscitation summary

Unconscious baby

⬇

Airway open

⬇

No breathing

⬇

Send helper to

📞 **CALL AN AMBULANCE**

⬇

**Give five initial rescue breaths**

⬇

Begin CPR (30 chest compressions alternating with 2 rescue breaths)

⬇

Repeat for 1 minute

⬇

If not already done,

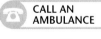
📞 **CALL AN AMBULANCE**

⬇

Continue CPR until help arrives

---

**❗ IMPORTANT**

● **If** you are unable or unwilling to give rescue breaths you can give chest compressions only.

---

# Rescue breathing: baby

This is to be used for an unconscious baby who is not breathing. Always give five initial rescue breaths before beginning chest compressions.

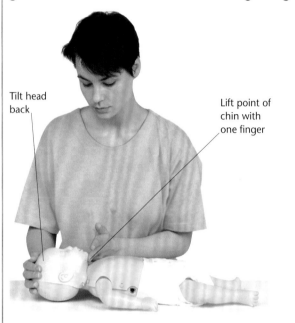

Tilt head back

Lift point of chin with one finger

**1** Make sure that her airway is open. Put your fingers on the point of the chin and lift it. Take care not to press on the soft part of the neck under the chin as that can block the airway.

Pick out visible obstructions

**2** Pick out any visible obstruction from the mouth and nose with your fingertips.

Blow into the baby's mouth and nose

**3** Take a breath, then seal your lips tightly around your baby's mouth and nose. Blow gently until the baby's chest rises.

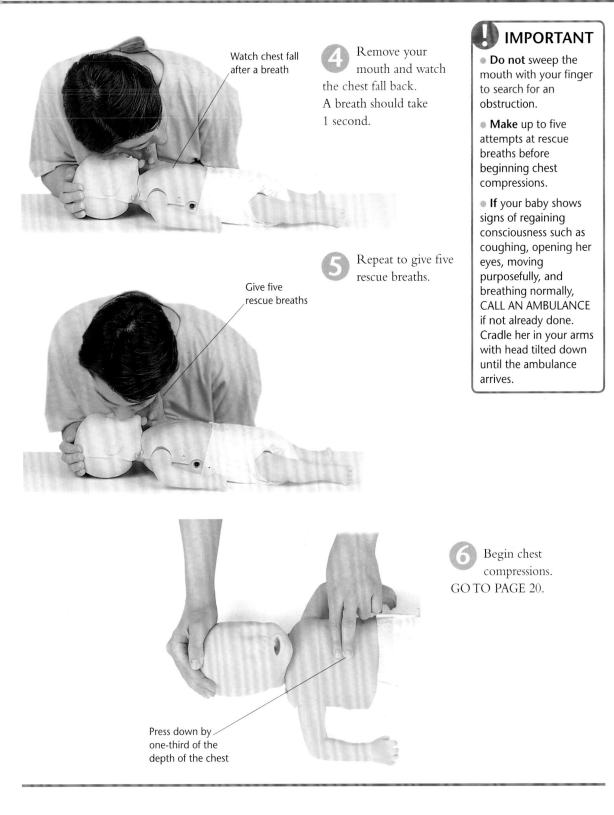

Watch chest fall
after a breath

**4** Remove your
mouth and watch
the chest fall back.
A breath should take
1 second.

**5** Repeat to give five
rescue breaths.

Give five
rescue breaths

**6** Begin chest
compressions.
GO TO PAGE 20.

Press down by
one-third of the
depth of the chest

**!  IMPORTANT**

● **Do not** sweep the
mouth with your finger
to search for an
obstruction.

● **Make** up to five
attempts at rescue
breaths before
beginning chest
compressions.

● **If** your baby shows
signs of regaining
consciousness such as
coughing, opening her
eyes, moving
purposefully, and
breathing normally,
CALL AN AMBULANCE
if not already done.
Cradle her in your arms
with head tilted down
until the ambulance
arrives.

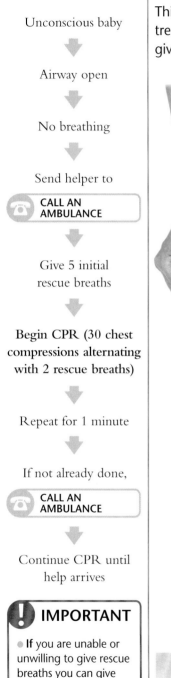

Unconscious baby

⬇

Airway open

⬇

No breathing

⬇

Send helper to

📞 CALL AN AMBULANCE

⬇

Give 5 initial rescue breaths

⬇

**Begin CPR (30 chest compressions alternating with 2 rescue breaths)**

⬇

Repeat for 1 minute

⬇

If not already done,

📞 CALL AN AMBULANCE

⬇

Continue CPR until help arrives

⚠ **IMPORTANT**

● If you are unable or unwilling to give rescue breaths you can give chest compressions only.

# CPR: baby

This is a combination of chest compressions and rescue breaths used to treat an unconscious baby who is not breathing. If you are on your own give CPR for one minute before you call an ambulance.

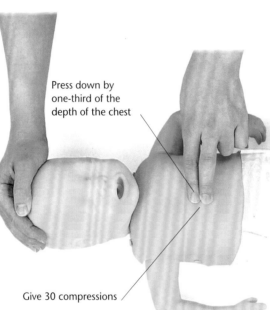

Press down by one-third of the depth of the chest

Give 30 compressions

**1** Place the tips of two fingers on the centre of the baby's chest.

**2** Press down firmly by one-third of the depth of the chest. Release the pressure but do not remove your fingers. Allow chest to come back up fully. Repeat to give 30 compressions at a rate of 100–120 per minute.

**3** Give your baby two rescue breaths into her mouth and nose.

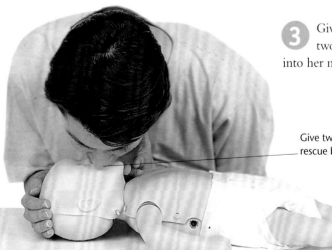

Give two rescue breaths

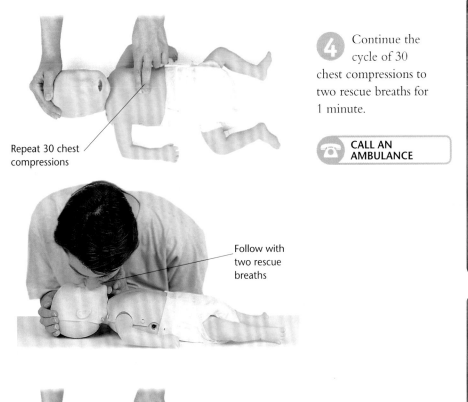

Repeat 30 chest compressions

**4** Continue the cycle of 30 chest compressions to two rescue breaths for 1 minute.

☎ **CALL AN AMBULANCE**

Follow with two rescue breaths

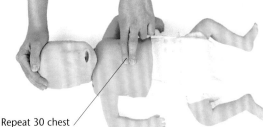

Repeat 30 chest compressions

**5** Continue giving CPR – 30 chest compressions followed by two rescue breaths – until emergency help arrives, or the baby shows signs of regaining consciousness.

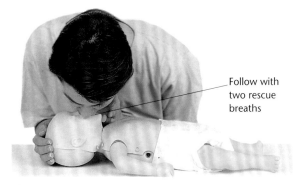

Follow with two rescue breaths

## ❗ IMPORTANT

● **If** your baby shows signs of regaining consciousness such as coughing, opening her eyes, moving purposefully, and breathing normally, CALL AN AMBULANCE if not already done. Cradle her in your arms with head tilted down until the ambulance arrives.

● **Take** your baby with you when you go to call the ambulance.

## The recovery position

Hold the baby in your arms with her head tilted downwards and supported. This keeps her air passages open and allows fluid to drain away.

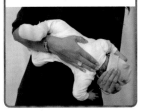

## ⟫ *see also*
● Rescue breathing: baby, *p.18*

## Resuscitation summary

**Unconscious child**

**Airway open**

↓

**No breathing**

↓

**Send helper to**

📞 **CALL AN AMBULANCE**

↓

Give five initial rescue breaths

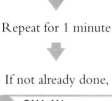

Begin CPR (30 chest compressions alternating with 2 rescue breaths)

Repeat for 1 minute

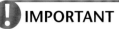

If not already done,

📞 **CALL AN AMBULANCE**

↓

Continue CPR until help arrives

> ❗ **IMPORTANT**
> ● **If** you are unable or unwilling to give rescue breaths you can give chest compressions only.

# Unconscious child

Assess your child before calling for help. If you are on your own and the child is not breathing, begin rescue breaths and chest compressions.

## ① Check for response

- Call his name, or tap his shoulder gently. Never shake a child.
- If there is no response, go to step 2.
- If there is a response,

🔖 **SEEK MEDICAL ADVICE**

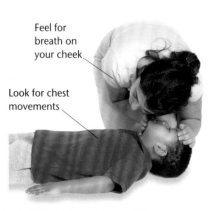

Tap his shoulder gently

## ② Open child's airway

- Put one hand on the child's forehead and gently tilt his head back.
- Place two fingers of your other hand on the tip of his chin and lift it.

> ❗ **IMPORTANT**
> ● **Do not** press the soft part of the neck under the chin as it can block the airway.

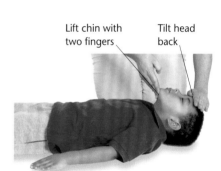

Lift chin with two fingers

Tilt head back

## ③ Check breathing for up to 10 seconds

- Look, listen, and feel for breathing. Look along his chest for movement, listen for sounds of breathing, and feel for breaths against your cheek. Send a helper to:

📞 **CALL AN AMBULANCE**

- If he is breathing place him in the recovery position. GO TO PAGE 28.
- If he not breathing, begin rescue breaths. GO TO PAGE 24.

Feel for breath on your cheek

Look for chest movements

# Using an AED on a child

Machines called AEDs (automated external defibrillators) can be used to analyse the heart rhythm and if necessary restart the heart. If a child is unconscious and not breathing, start rescue breaths and chest compressions (CPR, *see pp.24–27*), CALL AN AMBULANCE and request an AED. If there is an AED available, use it as soon as it arrives. The machine will give you a series of audible prompts to follow. If a shock is needed the machine will deliver it; if it is not needed it also knows not to deliver one.

**1** Put the AED beside the child, open the lid and take out the electrode pads – they will be attached to the machine.

**2** Place the pads on the child's chest. Peel off the backing paper and put one on the upper right side of the child's chest and the other on her lower left side.

**3** Once the pads are attached, make sure no-one is touching the child. The AED will analyse the heart rhythm and may recommend delivering a shock. Listen to the machine's instructions.

### IF A SHOCK IS ADVISED
- The AED will start to charge up – make sure everyone is clear of the child, then push the shock button when the AED gives the instruction.
- Continue CPR until the machine asks you to stop.
- The AED will re-analyse the child's heart rhythm at regular intervals.

### IF A SHOCK IS NOT ADVISED
- Continue CPR. The AED will re-analyse the child's heart rhythm at regular intervals.

Place one pad on left side of chest so that long axis is vertical

AED

Place one pad on upper right side of chest

Ask all helpers to stay clear of the child during analysis and shock

---

### ❗ IMPORTANT

- **If** a child's AED is not available, you can use an adult machine for a child aged 1–8. Ideally use paediatric pads.

- **Do not** use an AED on a baby under the age of one year.

- **If** the child is very small, place one pad in the centre of her back and the other one in the centre of the chest. Both pads should be vertical.

- **If** she starts coughing, opening her eyes, speaking or moving purposefully, and breathing normally, leave pads attached and put her in the recovery position.

## Resuscitation summary

Unconscious child

⬇

Airway open

⬇

No breathing

⬇

Send helper to

☎ **CALL AN AMBULANCE**

⬇

**Give five initial rescue breaths**

⬇

Begin CPR (30 chest compressions alternating with 2 rescue breaths)

⬇

Repeat for 1 minute

⬇

If not already done,

☎ **CALL AN AMBULANCE**

⬇

Continue CPR until help arrives

**❗ IMPORTANT**

● **If** you are unable or unwilling to give rescue breaths you can give chest compressions only.

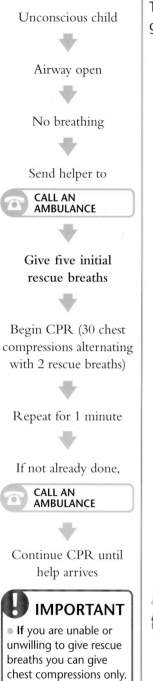

# Rescue breathing: child

This is to be used for an unconscious child who is not breathing. Always give five initial rescue breaths before beginning chest compressions.

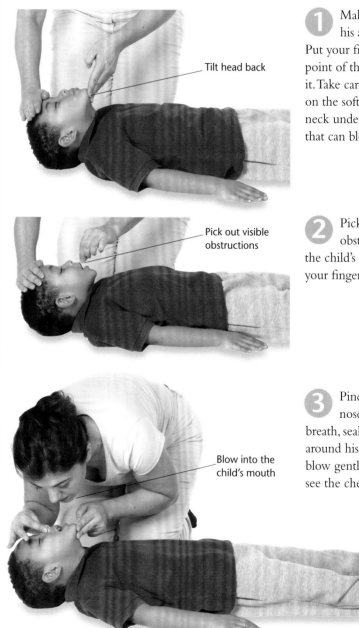

Tilt head back

**1** Make sure that his airway is open. Put your fingers on the point of the chin and lift it. Take care not to press on the soft part of the neck under the chin, as that can block the airway.

Pick out visible obstructions

**2** Pick out any visible obstructions from the child's mouth with your fingertips.

Blow into the child's mouth

**3** Pinch the child's nose. Take a breath, seal your lips around his mouth and blow gently until you see the chest rise.

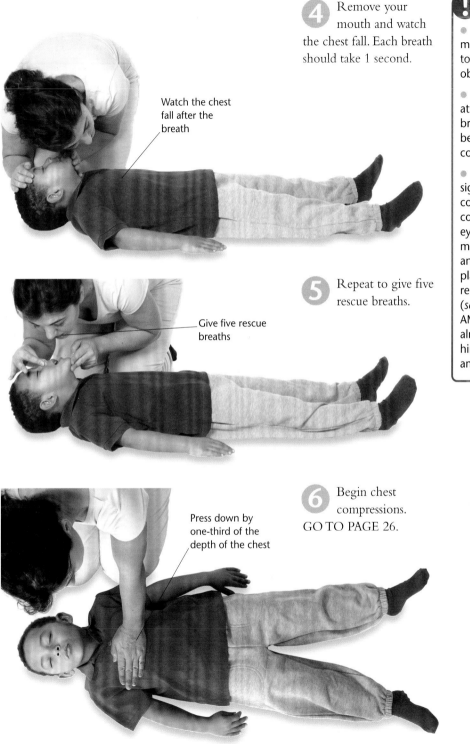

**4** Remove your mouth and watch the chest fall. Each breath should take 1 second.

Watch the chest fall after the breath

**5** Repeat to give five rescue breaths.

Give five rescue breaths

**6** Begin chest compressions. GO TO PAGE 26.

Press down by one-third of the depth of the chest

## ! IMPORTANT

● **Do not** sweep the mouth with your finger to search for an obstruction.

● **Make** up to five attempts at rescue breaths before beginning chest compressions.

● **If** your child shows signs of regaining consciousness such as coughing, opening his eyes, speaking or moving purposefully, and breathing normally, place him in the recovery position (*see p.28*) and CALL AN AMBULANCE if not already done. Monitor him carefully until the ambulance arrives.

# CPR: child

This is a combination of chest compressions and rescue breaths used to treat an unconscious child who is not breathing. If you are alone, give CPR for one minute before you call an ambulance.

## Resuscitation summary

Unconscious child

⬇

Airway open

⬇

No breathing

⬇

Send helper to

☎ **CALL AN AMBULANCE**

⬇

Give five initial rescue breaths

⬇

**Begin CPR (30 chest compressions alternating with 2 rescue breaths)**

⬇

Repeat for 1 minute

⬇

If not already done,

☎ **CALL AN AMBULANCE**

⬇

Continue CPR until help arrives

! **IMPORTANT**

- **If you are unable or unwilling to give rescue breaths you can give chest compressions only.**

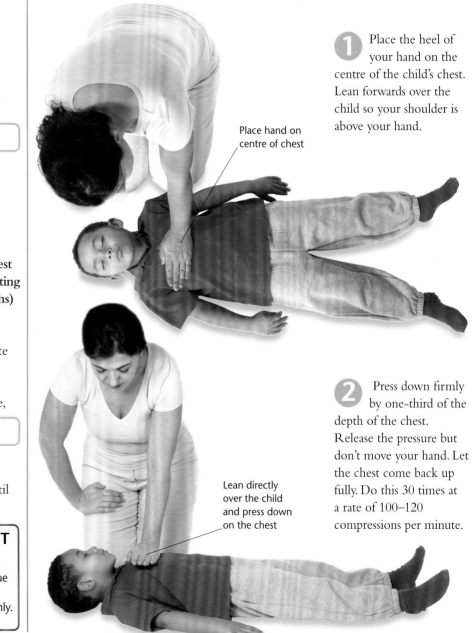

Place hand on centre of chest

**1** Place the heel of your hand on the centre of the child's chest. Lean forwards over the child so your shoulder is above your hand.

Lean directly over the child and press down on the chest

**2** Press down firmly by one-third of the depth of the chest. Release the pressure but don't move your hand. Let the chest come back up fully. Do this 30 times at a rate of 100–120 compressions per minute.

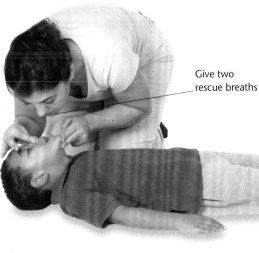

Give two rescue breaths

**3** Tilt the child's head back, lift the chin, and give TWO rescue breaths (*see p.24*).

**4** Continue the CPR cycle of 30 chest compressions to two rescue breaths for 1 minute. Then if not already done,

☎ **CALL AN AMBULANCE**

**‼ IMPORTANT**

● **If** your child shows signs of regaining consciousness such as coughing, opening his eyes, speaking or moving purposefully, and breathing normally, place him in the recovery position (*see p.28*) and CALL AN AMBULANCE if not already done. Monitor him carefully until the ambulance arrives.

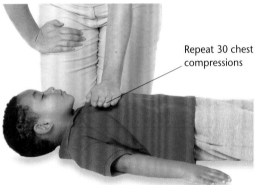

Repeat 30 chest compressions

**5** Continue giving CPR – 30 chest compressions followed by two rescue breaths – until emergency help arrives, or the child shows signs of regaining consciousness.

## For a larger child or small rescuer

If the child is large, or you are small, you can deliver chest compressions with two hands. Place one hand on the centre of the child's chest, then put your other hand on top and interlock your fingers. Then press down firmly.

Interlock your fingers

Keep your fingers off the child's chest

# Recovery position

Put your child in this position if she is unconscious but breathing to prevent her choking on her tongue or vomit.

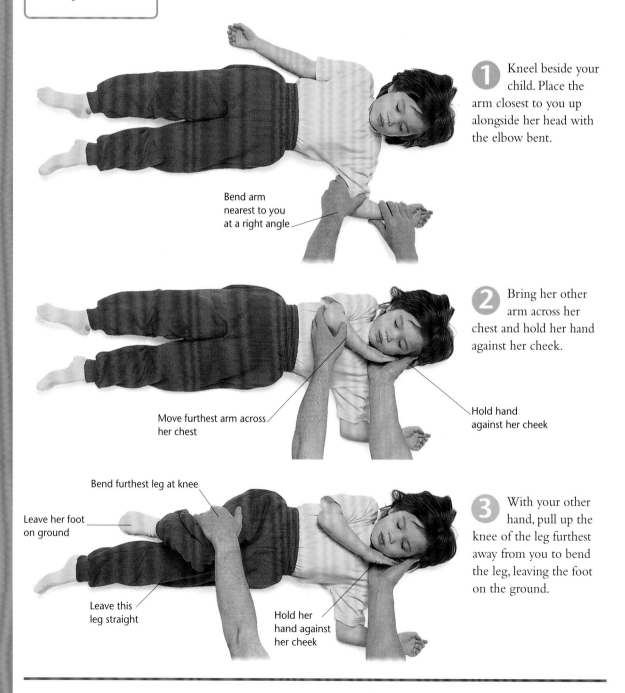

**1** Kneel beside your child. Place the arm closest to you up alongside her head with the elbow bent.

Bend arm nearest to you at a right angle

**2** Bring her other arm across her chest and hold her hand against her cheek.

Move furthest arm across her chest

Hold hand against her cheek

Bend furthest leg at knee

Leave her foot on ground

**3** With your other hand, pull up the knee of the leg furthest away from you to bend the leg, leaving the foot on the ground.

Leave this leg straight

Hold her hand against her cheek

**4** Pull the bent leg towards you to roll your child onto her side. Keep your child's hand against her cheek to support her head.

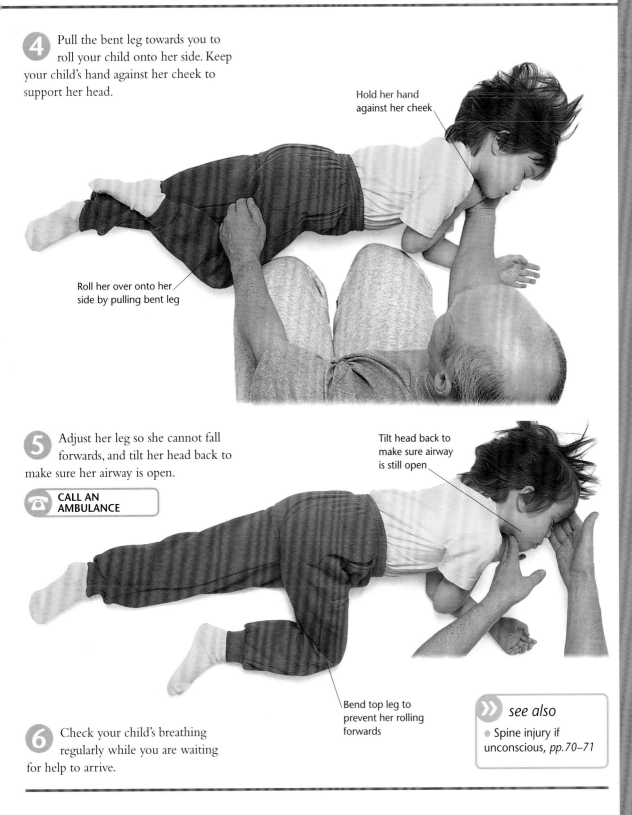

Hold her hand against her cheek

Roll her over onto her side by pulling bent leg

**5** Adjust her leg so she cannot fall forwards, and tilt her head back to make sure her airway is open.

**CALL AN AMBULANCE**

Tilt head back to make sure airway is still open

Bend top leg to prevent her rolling forwards

**6** Check your child's breathing regularly while you are waiting for help to arrive.

**»** *see also*
- Spine injury if unconscious, *pp.70–71*

## ! IMPORTANT

● **Do not** move your child unnecessarily.

● **Do not** give your child anything to drink or eat. If he is thirsty, just moisten his lips with water.

● **Do not** to leave a child in shock alone. If you can, send someone else to telephone for the ambulance while you stay with him.

# Shock

The most likely cause of shock is serious bleeding or a severe burn or scald. These injuries must be treated without delay. There could be internal bleeding if there are signs of shock and no visible injury. Early signs are: pale, cold, and sweaty skin, tinged with grey; rapid pulse becoming weaker; shallow, fast breathing. As it develops you will notice: restlessness; yawning and sighing; severe thirst; then unconsciousness.

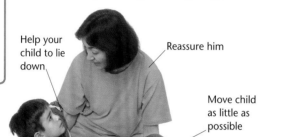

Help your child to lie down

Reassure him

Move child as little as possible

1 Help your child to lie down flat, on a blanket or rug if possible to protect him from the cold. Stay calm and reassure him. Treat any injury found.

☎ CALL AN AMBULANCE

2 Keep your child's head lower than his chest. Carefully raise your child's legs to help blood flow to the heart; support them on pillows, a chair, or a pile of books padded with a cushion.

Head must be lower than his chest

Raise his legs high above level of his heart

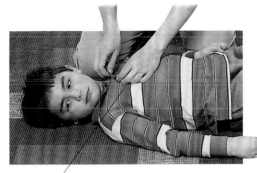

**3** To make breathing easier, loosen any fastenings or tight clothing at his neck, chest, and waist.

Loosen any tight clothing

**4** Put a blanket or coat over your child to keep him warm. DO NOT give him a hot-water bottle or apply any other source of direct heat; it can draw blood away from the heart.

Reassure your child

Cover him to keep him warm

> **! IMPORTANT**
>
> ● If your child loses consciousness, open his airway and check breathing. If breathing, place him in the recovery position; if not breathing, begin rescue breaths and chest compressions.

Observe and monitor his pulse, breathing rate, and level of consciousness

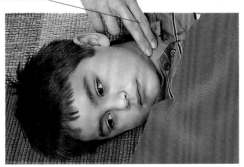

**5** Monitor his pulse, breathing rate, and level of consciousness while you wait for the ambulance. Encourage him to talk or answer questions. This will help you assess any change in his condition. Note any changes and tell the ambulance personnel.

> **》 see also**
>
> ● Bleeding, *p.44*
>
> ● Burns and scalds, *p.58*
>
> ● Unconscious baby, *pp.17–21*
>
> ● Unconscious child, *pp.22–29*

# Febrile seizures

Young children may develop these seizures when they have a high temperature. Suspect a possible febrile seizure if: your child is flushed and sweating with a very hot forehead; her eyes are rolled upwards, and possibly fixed or squinting; she is holding her breath and her face looks blue; she stiffens, arches her back and clenches her fists.

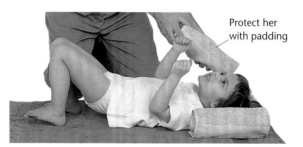

Protect her with padding

**1** Place soft padding, such as towels or pillows, around your child so that even violent movement will not lead to injury.

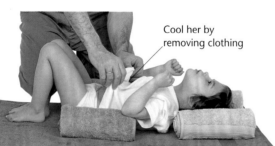

Cool her by removing clothing

**2** Undress your child to help cool her down. Make sure there is a good supply of cool fresh air, but be careful not to overcool her.

After seizure stops, cover her with a sheet

Place her in recovery position

**3** Seizures will stop when your child is cooled. Place her in the recovery position. Cover her with a light blanket or sheet and reassure her. If her temperature rises again, repeat steps 1 and 2.

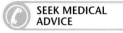

**SEEK MEDICAL ADVICE**

**see also**

● Fever, *p.96*

● Unconscious baby, *pp.17–21*

● Unconscious child, *pp.22–29*

# Epileptic seizures

These are caused by a disturbance in the electrical activity of the brain. A seizure may progress through stages: sudden unconsciousness, sometimes with a cry; rigidity and arching of back; breathing may cease; jerking movements begin; froth or bubbles appear at the mouth, possibly blood stained; loss of bladder or bowel control. The child regains consciousness within a few minutes and appears dazed. Afterwards she may fall into a deep sleep.

Clear away nearby objects, such as chairs

**1** If your child starts to fall, help her to the floor. Prevent injury by clearing away objects that she may knock against.

**2** Place padding under or around her head to prevent injury.

**3** When her seizure is over, your child may be unconscious. Remove any padding and open her airway and check breathing.

Protect her head with soft padding

Place her in the recovery position if breathing

**4** If she is breathing, place her in the recovery position. Stay with her until she is recovered. She may feel dazed and behave oddly, or sleep deeply.

SEEK MEDICAL ADVICE

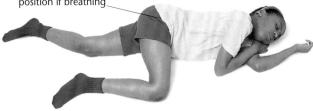

## IMPORTANT

● **Look** for a card or bracelet alerting you to the fact that a child has a history of epilepsy.

● **Do not** hold her down or try to move her during the seizure.

● **Do not** put anything in her mouth or give her anything to eat or drink.

● **If** your child has never had a seizure before, a seizure lasts more than 5 minutes, if she has repeated seizures, or if she is unconscious for more than 10 minutes CALL AN AMBULANCE.

## Absence seizures

These seizures can be recognised by a momentary "switching off", some facial twitching, or distracted movements such as lip-smacking. If this happens, reassure the child and SEEK MEDICAL ADVICE.

## see also

● Unconscious baby, *pp.17–21*

● Unconscious child, *pp.22–29*

# Diabetic emergency

If a child with diabetes has low blood sugar levels he will be: weak or hungry; confused or behave aggressively; sweating; very pale. He may also have a strong, bounding pulse and breathing may be shallow.

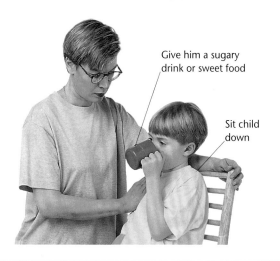

Give him a sugary drink or sweet food

Sit child down

**1** Help your child to sit down and give him a sweet drink or food to raise blood sugar levels.

**2** If he improves rapidly after a sweet drink or food, give him some more and let him rest.

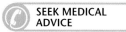
**SEEK MEDICAL ADVICE**

## If the child is unconscious

If a child with diabetes is unconscious, **do not** offer her anything to eat or drink.

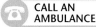
**CALL AN AMBULANCE**

**1** Open the airway and check breathing.

**2** If she is breathing, place her in the recovery position.

**3** If she is not breathing, begin rescue breaths and chest compressions.

Open airway

Check for breathing

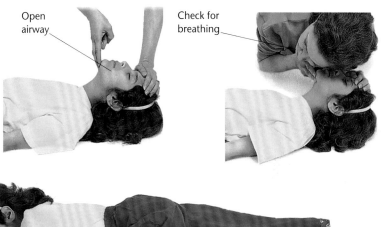

Place breathing child in the recovery position

# Faint

Your child may be about to faint if she complains of feeling weak, giddy and sick, and is very pale. Loss of consciousness is brief and accompanied by a very slow pulse; recovery is rapid and complete.

**1** Help your child to lie down and raise her legs above the level of her heart; this improves the blood flow to her brain. Support her legs on a pile of cushions or folded blankets.

**2** Give her plenty of fresh air. If you are inside open a window. It can help to fan her face to circulate the air. Reassure your child and help her to sit her up gradually.

**!** **IMPORTANT**

● **Do not** sit your child on a chair with her head down if she is feeling faint as she may fall and hurt herself.

● **If** your child is unconscious, open her airway and check breathing. If breathing, place in the recovery position; if not breathing, begin rescue breaths and chest compressions. CALL AN AMBULANCE.

**»** *see also*

● Unconscious child, *pp.22–29*

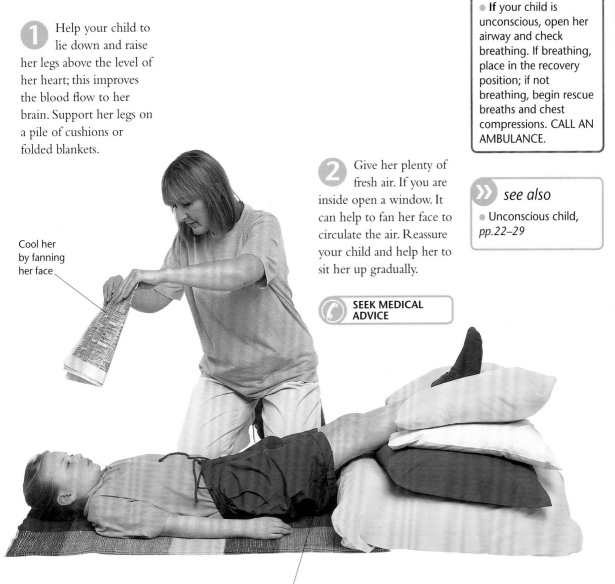

Cool her by fanning her face

**SEEK MEDICAL ADVICE**

Raise her legs above the level of her heart

# Choking baby

If the choking is mild, your baby will still be able to cough, and cry. If the blockage is severe, however, he will be unable to cry, cough, or breathe. Give back blows then chest thrusts to relieve the blockage.

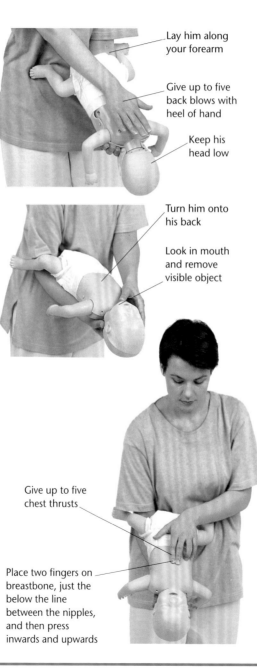

Lay him along your forearm

Give up to five back blows with heel of hand

Keep his head low

Turn him onto his back

Look in mouth and remove visible object

Give up to five chest thrusts

Place two fingers on breastbone, just the below the line between the nipples, and then press inwards and upwards

**1** If your baby is unable to cough or breathe, lay him face down, head lower than his bottom, along your forearm. Support his head and shoulders with your hand. Give up to five back blows with the heel of your hand.

**2** Turn him face up along your other arm. Pick out any visible obstruction from the mouth or nose with your fingertips.

**3** If the obstruction has not cleared, give up to five chest thrusts. Place two fingers on the lower half of the baby's breastbone and push inwards and upwards towards his head. Then check his mouth.

**4** If the obstruction still has not cleared, repeat steps 1–3 three times.

☎ **CALL AN AMBULANCE**

**5** Continue cycles of back blows and chest thrusts until help arrives, the obstruction clears, or the baby loses consciousness.

# If your baby becomes unconscious

If your baby loses consciousness, begin CPR. If he starts breathing at any stage, cradle him in your arms with his head tilted down in the baby recovery position (*see p.21*).

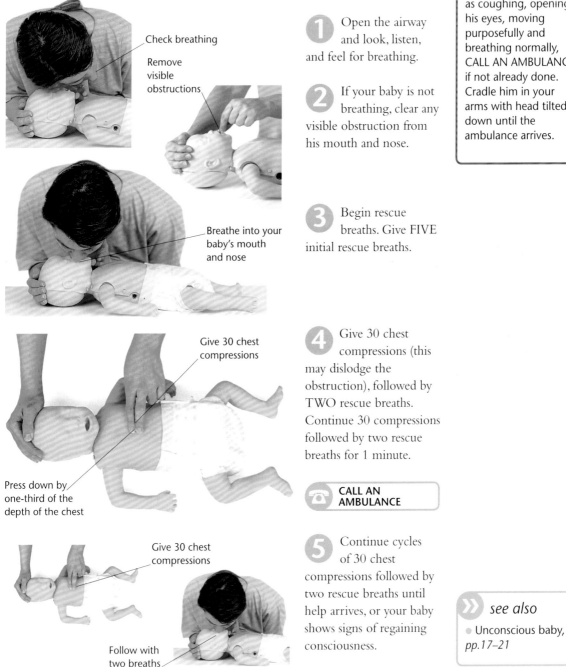

Check breathing

Remove visible obstructions

Breathe into your baby's mouth and nose

Give 30 chest compressions

Press down by one-third of the depth of the chest

Give 30 chest compressions

Follow with two breaths

**1** Open the airway and look, listen, and feel for breathing.

**2** If your baby is not breathing, clear any visible obstruction from his mouth and nose.

**3** Begin rescue breaths. Give FIVE initial rescue breaths.

**4** Give 30 chest compressions (this may dislodge the obstruction), followed by TWO rescue breaths. Continue 30 compressions followed by two rescue breaths for 1 minute.

**☎ CALL AN AMBULANCE**

**5** Continue cycles of 30 chest compressions followed by two rescue breaths until help arrives, or your baby shows signs of regaining consciousness.

**》 see also**
● Unconscious baby, *pp.17–21*

# Choking child

Start by asking your child if he is choking. If the blockage is mild, he will be able to speak, cough, and breathe. If it is severe, he will not be able to speak, cough, or breathe.

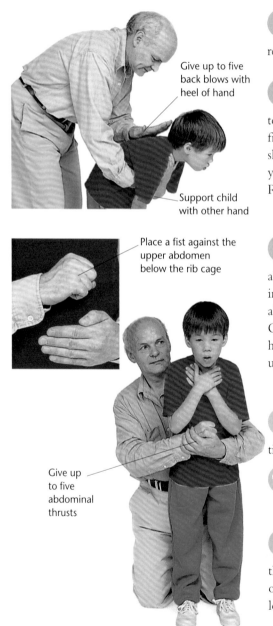

Give up to five back blows with heel of hand

Support child with other hand

Place a fist against the upper abdomen below the rib cage

Give up to five abdominal thrusts

**1** If your child can cough, encourage him to do so to remove the object.

**2** If your child cannot talk, cough, or breathe, help him to bend forwards. Give him up to five back blows between the shoulder blades with the heel of your hand.  Check his mouth. Remove any object you can see.

**3** If the obstruction has not cleared, give up to five abdominal thrusts. Place your fist in the middle of his upper abdomen, just below his rib cage. Cover the fist with your other hand and pull sharply inwards and upwards. Check his mouth.

**4** If the abdominal thrusts fail, repeat steps 2 and 3 three times. If this is unsuccessful,

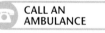
**CALL AN AMBULANCE**

**5** Continue cycles of back blows and abdominal thrusts until help arrives, the obstruction clears, or the child loses consciousness.

# If your child becomes unconscious

If your choking child loses consciousness treat as here. If he starts breathing at any stage, place him in the recovery position and SEEK MEDICAL ADVICE.

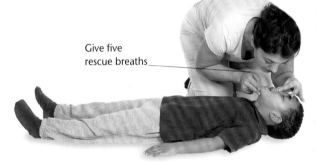

Tilt head to open airway

**1** Open his airway. Look, listen, and feel for breathing. If your child is not breathing, clear any visible obstruction from his mouth.

**2** Begin rescue breaths. Give FIVE initial rescue breaths.

Give five rescue breaths

**3** Give 30 chest compressions (this may dislodge obstruction), then repeat TWO rescue breaths. Continue to give 30 compressions followed by two rescue breaths for 1 minute.

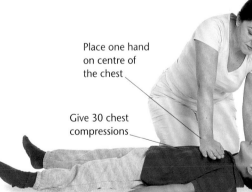

Place one hand on centre of the chest

Give 30 chest compressions

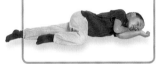
📞 **CALL AN AMBULANCE**

**4** Continue cycles of 30 chest compressions followed by two rescue breaths until help arrives, or your child shows signs of regaining consciousness.

## The recovery position

● **If** your child shows signs of regaining consciousness such as coughing, opening his eyes, speaking or moving purposefully, and breathing normally, place him in the recovery position (*see p.28*) and CALL AN AMBULANCE if not already done. Monitor him carefully until the ambulance arrives.

》 *see also*
● Unconscious child, *pp.22–29*

# Breath holding

This is the result of rage and frustration. Your child is breath holding if he cries, then breathes in but does not breathe out. He may go blue in the face and stiff and may even become unconscious momentarily.

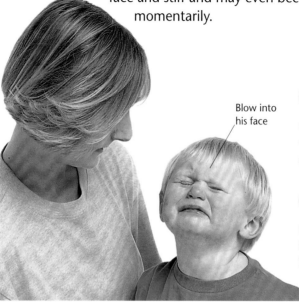

Blow into his face

**1** Try to stay calm. Do not shake him or make a fuss. He will usually start breathing again spontaneously.

**2** Try blowing directly into his face; this often results in a child starting to breathe again.

**»** *see also*

● Unconscious child, *pp.22–29*

# Hiccups

These are very common and usually only last for a few minutes, though often seem to go on for a long time. Children can become distressed.

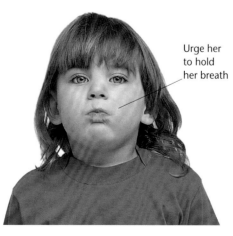

Urge her to hold her breath

**1** Tell your child to sit still and to hold her breath for as long as she can. Then encourage her to breathe out slowly.

**2** Get her to repeat this until hiccups have stopped.

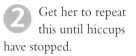

# Suffocation and strangulation

Strangulation results from a constriction around the child's neck that prevents breathing. Suffocation occurs when there is an obstruction over the mouth or nose, a weight on the child's chest or abdomen preventing normal breathing, or because the child is inhaling smoke- or fume-filled air, which prevents oxygen entering the lungs.

> **!  IMPORTANT**
>
> ● **If** your child is hanging, support his body while you remove or cut the rope or cord.
>
> ● **If** your child is not breathing, begin rescue breaths and chest compressions.

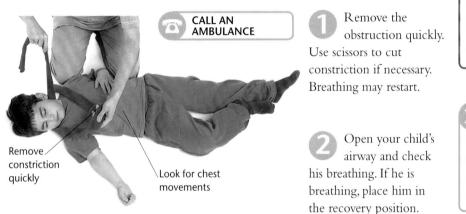

Remove constriction quickly

Look for chest movements

☎ **CALL AN AMBULANCE**

**1** Remove the obstruction quickly. Use scissors to cut constriction if necessary. Breathing may restart.

**2** Open your child's airway and check his breathing. If he is breathing, place him in the recovery position.

> **»  see also**
>
> ● Unconscious baby, pp.17–21
>
> ● Unconscious child, pp.22–29

# Fume inhalation

Fume, gas, and smoke inhalation requires urgent medical attention as the fumes prevent the child breathing in oxygen.

> **!  IMPORTANT**
>
> ● **Do not** enter the area if fumes, gas, or smoke are still present. CALL FIRE SERVICE and AMBULANCE.
>
> ● **If** your child is not breathing, begin rescue breaths and chest compressions.

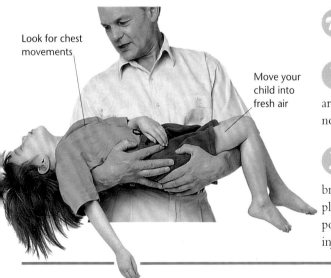

Look for chest movements

Move your child into fresh air

☎ **CALL AN AMBULANCE**

**1** Carry your child away from danger area. Ensure that you do not put yourself at risk.

**2** Open her airway and check her breathing. If breathing, place her in the recovery position, and treat any injuries found.

> **»  see also**
>
> ● Burns and scalds, p.58
>
> ● Unconscious baby, pp.17–21
>
> ● Unconscious child, pp.22–29

# Croup

This condition can be alarming and usually occurs at night, but passes quickly. Your child will have difficulty breathing, and a short, barking cough. He may be making a crowing or whistling noise. In a severe attack, he may use muscles around his nose, neck, and upper arms in his attempts to breathe and he may have blue-tinged skin.

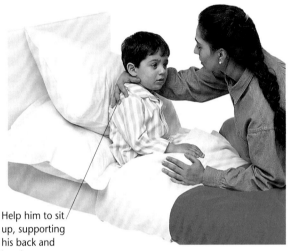

Help him to sit up, supporting his back and head

**1** Help your child to sit up in bed. Prop him up with pillows at his back and head and reassure him.

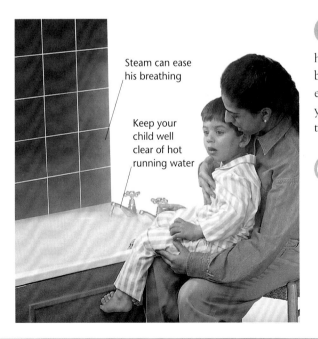

Steam can ease his breathing

Keep your child well clear of hot running water

**2** Create a steamy atmosphere; run hot water into the bath or boil a kettle in an enclosed room. Try to get your child to relax enough to breathe in the steam.

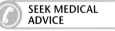
**SEEK MEDICAL ADVICE**

# Asthma

If your child suffers from asthma, familiarise her with her medication so that she knows how to use it in an attack. You can recognise an attack if your child: has difficulty breathing and is coughing; is wheezing especially when breathing *out;* is distressed and anxious. She may also be tired by efforts to breathe and have a bluish tinge to face and lips.

> ## ! IMPORTANT
> ● **If** it is a first attack, CALL AN AMBULANCE.
>
> ● **If** the attack is severe, the medication has no effect, the child is exhausted, or breathlessness makes talking difficult, CALL AN AMBULANCE.

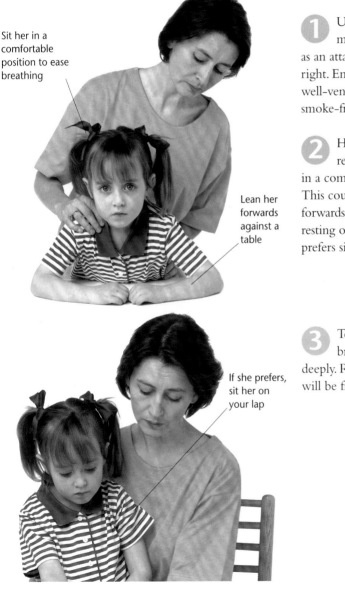

Sit her in a comfortable position to ease breathing

Lean her forwards against a table

If she prefers, sit her on your lap

**1** Use your child's medication as soon as an attack starts, see right. Ensure the room is well-ventilated and smoke-free.

**2** Help your child to relax. Sit her down in a comfortable position. This could be leaning forwards with her arms resting on a table, or if she prefers sit her on your lap.

**3** Tell her to try to breathe slowly and deeply. Reassure her as she will be frightened.

## Using medication

Use your child's medication as soon as an attack starts. Make sure you give her the reliever inhaler – this has a blue cap. Usually if a child has an inhaler she will also have a spacer device to use with it, so use that as well. Follow the directions carefully.

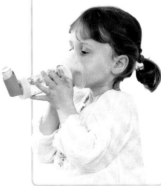

**!  IMPORTANT**

● **If** an object has become stuck in the wound, press either side of the object not directly over it.

● **If** blood comes through the first bandage, place another pad firmly on top and secure with a bandage. If blood continues to seep through dressings, pressure may not be in the right place. Remove both dressings and apply a new one, making sure pressure is over the wound.

● **If** the bleeding persists, follow the treatment for shock and CALL AN AMBULANCE.

# Bleeding

Severe bleeding can be distressing for you and your child. If it is not controlled your child may develop a life-threatening condition known as shock. Large wounds may need stitches.

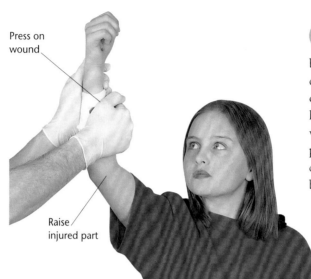

Press on wound

Raise injured part

**1** Press firmly on the wound to stop the bleeding. Press over a clean pad or handkerchief or put the palm of your hand directly on the wound. Raise the injured part above the level of the child's heart to reduce the blood flow to the injury.

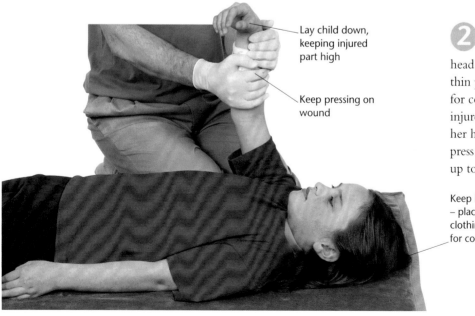

Lay child down, keeping injured part high

Keep pressing on wound

**2** Help your child to lie down, with her head low (you can put a thin pad under her head for comfort). Keep the injured part raised above her heart. Continue to press on the wound for up to 10 minutes.

Keep her head low – place a thin item of clothing under head for comfort

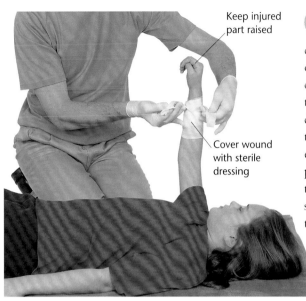

Keep injured part raised

Cover wound with sterile dressing

**3** Keeping the injured part raised, cover the wound and original pad with a sterile dressing that is larger than the wound. Secure the dressing with a bandage; the bandage must be firm enough to maintain pressure, but not so tight that it cuts off the blood supply to the area beyond the injury.

# When bleeding stops

Once the bleeding is under control, or stops, support the injury in a raised position – for example, with an elevation sling, *see p.107.* TAKE YOUR CHILD TO HOSPITAL.

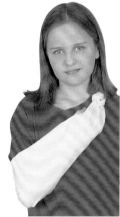

**4** If bleeding is still not under control, keep injury raised but in addition, elevate and support her legs so they are higher than her chest. Remove the clothing from under her head. Cover her to keep her warm. If she is thirsty, moisten her lips with water, but do not let her drink or eat.

📞 **CALL AN AMBULANCE**

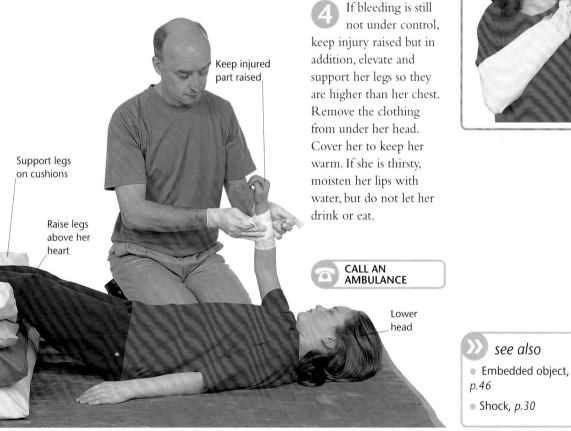

Keep injured part raised

Support legs on cushions

Raise legs above her heart

Lower head

>> *see also*
- Embedded object, *p.46*
- Shock, *p.30*

> **IMPORTANT**
● **Do not** try to remove, or dislodge, objects that are embedded in a wound as you may cause further damage and bleeding.

# Embedded object

A large object such as a piece of glass that becomes stuck in a wound is serious – it may be plugging the wound, preventing bleeding. Do not remove it. Protect it with padding and bandages and get medical help.

## Bandaging around larger objects

If the object is very big, build up padding around it, then bandage above and below the object instead of over the top.

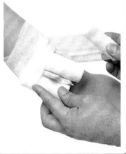

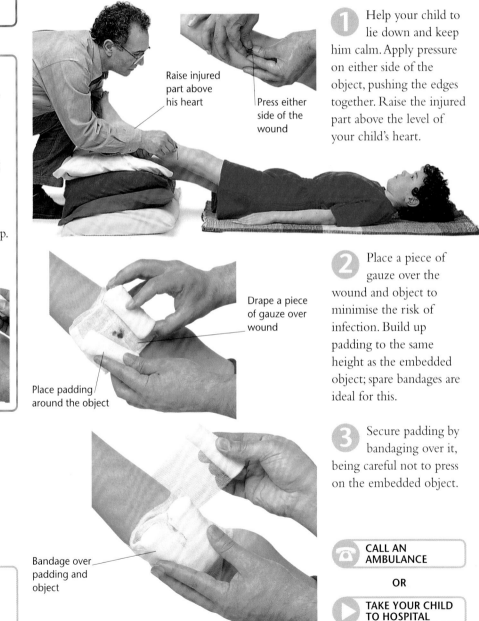

Raise injured part above his heart

Press either side of the wound

**1** Help your child to lie down and keep him calm. Apply pressure on either side of the object, pushing the edges together. Raise the injured part above the level of your child's heart.

Drape a piece of gauze over wound

Place padding around the object

**2** Place a piece of gauze over the wound and object to minimise the risk of infection. Build up padding to the same height as the embedded object; spare bandages are ideal for this.

**3** Secure padding by bandaging over it, being careful not to press on the embedded object.

Bandage over padding and object

☎ **CALL AN AMBULANCE**

**OR**

▶ **TAKE YOUR CHILD TO HOSPITAL**

>> *see also*
● Bleeding, *p.44*

# Cuts and grazes

Children can be very upset by the tiniest graze. Ressure your child and wash the wound. Covering the wound with a plaster keeps it clean and often makes the child feel better.

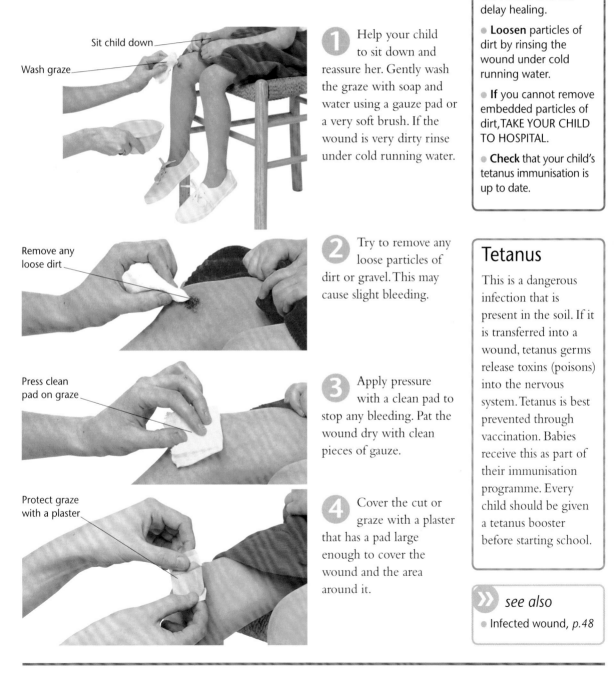

Sit child down

Wash graze

**1** Help your child to sit down and reassure her. Gently wash the graze with soap and water using a gauze pad or a very soft brush. If the wound is very dirty rinse under cold running water.

Remove any loose dirt

**2** Try to remove any loose particles of dirt or gravel. This may cause slight bleeding.

Press clean pad on graze

**3** Apply pressure with a clean pad to stop any bleeding. Pat the wound dry with clean pieces of gauze.

Protect graze with a plaster

**4** Cover the cut or graze with a plaster that has a pad large enough to cover the wound and the area around it.

---

**!** **IMPORTANT**

- **Do not** clean or cover cuts with cotton wool or any fluffy material; it may stick to the wound and will delay healing.

- **Loosen** particles of dirt by rinsing the wound under cold running water.

- **If** you cannot remove embedded particles of dirt, TAKE YOUR CHILD TO HOSPITAL.

- **Check** that your child's tetanus immunisation is up to date.

## Tetanus

This is a dangerous infection that is present in the soil. If it is transferred into a wound, tetanus germs release toxins (poisons) into the nervous system. Tetanus is best prevented through vaccination. Babies receive this as part of their immunisation programme. Every child should be given a tetanus booster before starting school.

**»** *see also*

- Infected wound, *p.48*

## ! IMPORTANT

● **Do not** try to remove objects that are embedded in a wound as you may cause further damage and bleeding.

## Tetanus

This is a dangerous infection that is present in the soil. If it is transferred into a wound, tetanus germs release toxins (poisons) into the nervous system. Tetanus is best prevented through vaccination. Babies receive this as part of their immunisation programme. Every child should be given a tetanus booster before starting school.

# Infected wound

A wound is infected if there is: increasing pain and soreness; swelling, redness, and a feeling of heat around the injury; pus within, or oozing from, the wound; swelling and tenderness in the glands in the neck, armpit, or groin; and possible faint red trails on the skin leading to these glands. When infection is advanced there may also be signs of fever (sweating, thirst, shivering, and lethargy).

Cover wound with a clean pad

**1** Cover the wound with a clean non-fluffy pad or sterile dressing secured in place with a bandage.

Bandage dressing in place

**2** Raise the infected wound, and support it, for example, with an elevation sling.

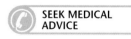

**SEEK MEDICAL ADVICE**

Raise and support injury

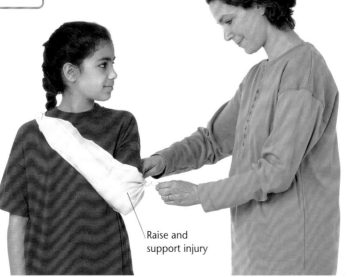

» *see also*
● Triangular bandages, *p.106*

# Blisters

If a blister is caused by friction (for example, a badly fitting shoe) treat as here. You can buy special padded blister plasters.

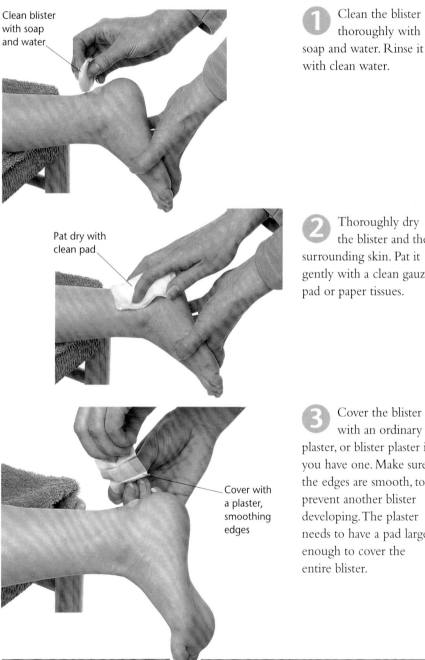

Clean blister with soap and water

**1** Clean the blister thoroughly with soap and water. Rinse it with clean water.

Pat dry with clean pad

**2** Thoroughly dry the blister and the surrounding skin. Pat it gently with a clean gauze pad or paper tissues.

Cover with a plaster, smoothing edges

**3** Cover the blister with an ordinary plaster, or blister plaster if you have one. Make sure the edges are smooth, to prevent another blister developing. The plaster needs to have a pad large enough to cover the entire blister.

>> *see also*
● Burns and scalds, p.58

# Eye wound

This type of wound is serious because of the risk of damage to the child's sight. Injury can scar the surface of the eye or lead to infection.

> ! **IMPORTANT**
> ● **Do not** try to remove objects in the eye.
> ● **If** you cannot transport your child lying on his back, CALL AN AMBULANCE.

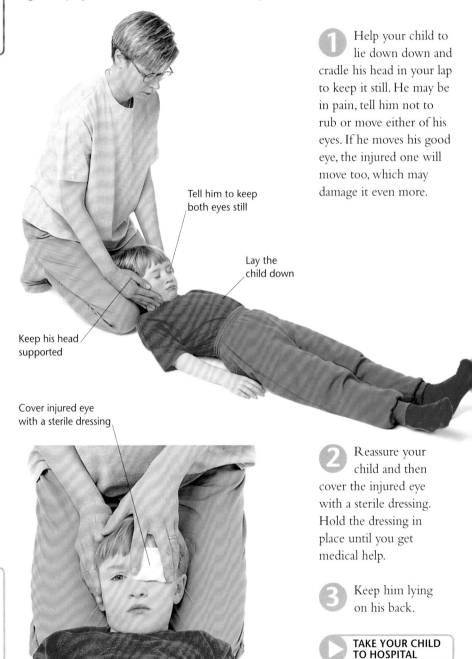

Tell him to keep both eyes still

Lay the child down

Keep his head supported

Cover injured eye with a sterile dressing

**1** Help your child to lie down down and cradle his head in your lap to keep it still. He may be in pain, tell him not to rub or move either of his eyes. If he moves his good eye, the injured one will move too, which may damage it even more.

**2** Reassure your child and then cover the injured eye with a sterile dressing. Hold the dressing in place until you get medical help.

**3** Keep him lying on his back.

> ▶ **TAKE YOUR CHILD TO HOSPITAL**

> ≫ *see also*
> ● Chemical burn to eye, *p.62*
> ● Object in eye, *p.82*

# Nosebleed

Children get nosebleeds from a blow to the nose, or from picking it. Bleeding usually stops quickly, but it can alarm young children.

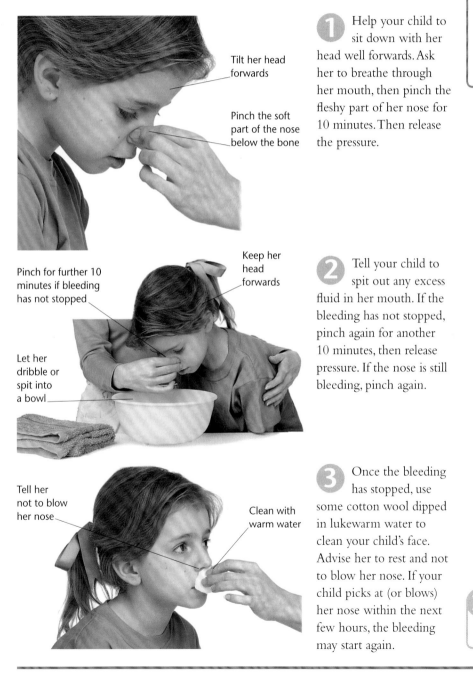

Tilt her head forwards

Pinch the soft part of the nose below the bone

**1** Help your child to sit down with her head well forwards. Ask her to breathe through her mouth, then pinch the fleshy part of her nose for 10 minutes. Then release the pressure.

Keep her head forwards

Pinch for further 10 minutes if bleeding has not stopped

Let her dribble or spit into a bowl

**2** Tell your child to spit out any excess fluid in her mouth. If the bleeding has not stopped, pinch again for another 10 minutes, then release pressure. If the nose is still bleeding, pinch again.

Tell her not to blow her nose

Clean with warm water

**3** Once the bleeding has stopped, use some cotton wool dipped in lukewarm water to clean your child's face. Advise her to rest and not to blow her nose. If your child picks at (or blows) her nose within the next few hours, the bleeding may start again.

**»  see also**
● Head injury, p.66

> **! IMPORTANT**
>
> ● **If** the bleeding follows a head injury and there is thin, watery fluid draining from the ear, CALL AN AMBULANCE.
>
> ● **If** the injury is caused by an earring being ripped out, your child may need stitches. TAKE YOUR CHILD TO HOSPITAL.

## Bleeding from inside the ear

Help your child into a semi-upright position, with his head tilted towards the injured side, to allow blood to drain away. Put an absorbent pad over the ear and bandage it lightly in place. Do not plug the ear. SEEK MEDICAL ADVICE.

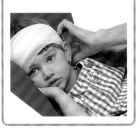

>> *see also*
● Object in ear, *p.83*
● Head injury, *p.66*

# Ear wound

Outer ear wounds can bleed profusely, which can be alarming. If blood is coming from inside the ear, check that your child has not inserted something into it. If bleeding follows a head injury, CALL AN AMBULANCE.

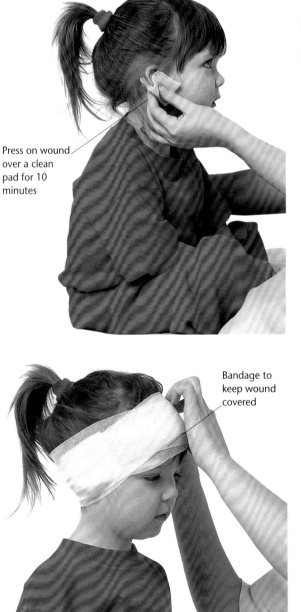

Press on wound over a clean pad for 10 minutes

Bandage to keep wound covered

**1** Help your child to sit down and gently pinch the wound with your thumb and forefinger over a clean piece of gauze. Keep pressing for 10 minutes.

**2** Cover the injured ear with a sterile dressing and lightly bandage it in place.

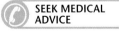 **SEEK MEDICAL ADVICE**

# Mouth wound

These wounds can be the result of a child biting the inside of his mouth in a fall, for example, or from the loss of a tooth. Make sure your child does not inhale blood, as this can result in breathing problems.

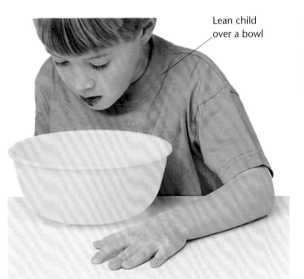

Lean child over a bowl

**1** Help your child to sit down with his head over a bowl. Encourage him to spit out any blood.

## Bleeding from tooth socket

Place a pad over the tooth socket, making sure that it is higher than the adjacent teeth so that your child can bite on it. Ask your child to sit down with her hand supporting her jaw. Tell her to bite hard on the pad. A younger child may need you to hold the pad in place.

Press on wound over a clean pad for 10 minutes

**2** Place a pad over the wound and pinch it between your thumb and forefinger, maintaining the pressure for 10 minutes. Your child may be able to do this for himself.

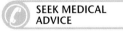

SEEK MEDICAL ADVICE

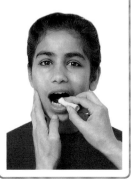

# Amputation

## Care of the amputated part

Wrap the severed part in kitchen film or a plastic bag. Wrap the bag in a soft fabric, such as a cotton handkerchief or piece of gauze. Put a plastic bag filled with ice cubes around the fabric. This helps preserve the severed part until you get to hospital. Put the whole package in another bag or container. Mark with the time of injury and the child's name and give it to the ambulance personnel.

Whether a injury causes partial or total amputation, the limb can often be reattached. Your child will need an anaesthetic so don't give him anything to eat or drink because it will delay surgery.

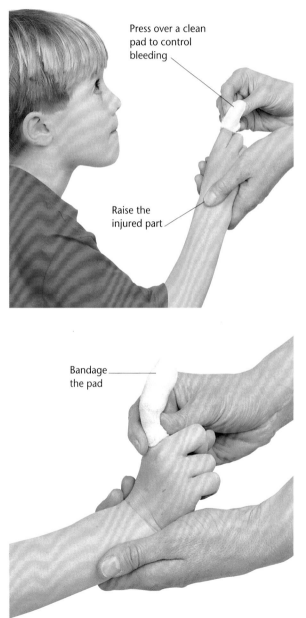

Press over a clean pad to control bleeding

Raise the injured part

Bandage the pad

**1** Control the blood loss by pressing firmly on the injury using a sterile dressing or clean pad. Raise the injured part above the level of your child's heart. If necessary, help your child to lie down and raise his legs above his heart.

**2** Bandage or tape the dressing firmly in place. You can cover a finger with a gauze finger bandage to protect it.

### ☎ CALL AN AMBULANCE

**3** Tell the ambulance control it is an amputation. Monitor your child for signs of shock while waiting. If possible, put the severed part in a plastic bag, see left.

### ≫ see also
● Bleeding, *p.44*
● Shock, *p.30*

# Internal bleeding

Suspect this when signs of shock develop without obvious blood loss. There may also be "pattern bruising" around the injury with marks from clothes or crushing objects. There could also be bleeding from orifices, such as the nose or ear. Note what this looks like and keep a sample.

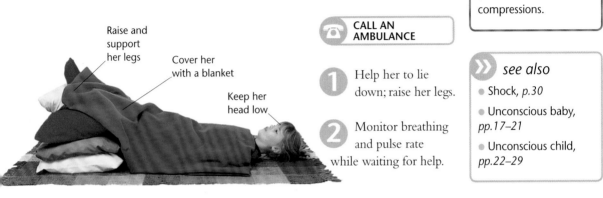

Raise and support her legs

Cover her with a blanket

Keep her head low

**IMPORTANT**

● **If** child is unconscious, open her airway and check breathing. If breathing, place in the recovery position; if not breathing, begin rescue breaths and chest compressions.

**CALL AN AMBULANCE**

**1** Help her to lie down; raise her legs.

**2** Monitor breathing and pulse rate while waiting for help.

**see also**

● Shock, *p.30*
● Unconscious baby, *pp.17–21*
● Unconscious child, *pp.22–29*

# Crush injury

A crush injury can be serious as it may cause internal bleeding and broken bones as well as open wounds.

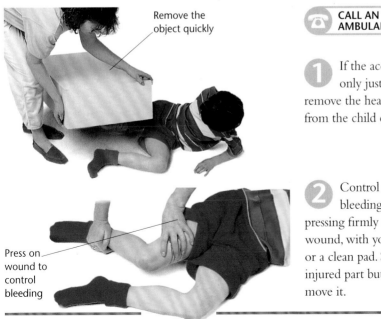

Remove the object quickly

Press on wound to control bleeding

**CALL AN AMBULANCE**

**1** If the accident has only just happened, remove the heavy object from the child quickly.

**2** Control any bleeding by pressing firmly on the wound, with your hand or a clean pad. Support the injured part but do not move it.

**IMPORTANT**

● **If** your child has been crushed for over 15 minutes, do not remove the object as it may cause toxic fluids from the damaged muscles to be released into the body. This increases the risk of shock which can be fatal.

● **If** you suspect broken bones, support the injury but do not move your child unless he is in immediate danger. Watch for signs of shock while waiting for help.

**see also**

● Bleeding, *p.44*
● Shock, *p.30*
● Broken bone, *p.72*

> **IMPORTANT**
● **Monitor** your child for signs of shock.

● **If** child loses consciousness, open his airway and check breathing. If breathing, place in the recovery position; if not breathing, begin rescue breaths and chest compressions.

# Chest wound

A chest wound may cause severe internal injuries. The lungs are particularly vulnerable, and breathing problems, shock, and collapsed lungs may follow an injury. It is important to make an airtight seal over the wound to prevent air entering the chest cavity.

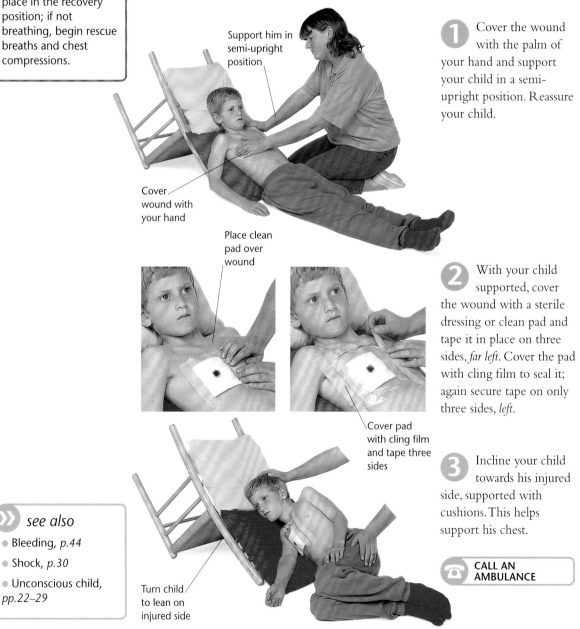

Support him in semi-upright position

Cover wound with your hand

Place clean pad over wound

Cover pad with cling film and tape three sides

Turn child to lean on injured side

**1** Cover the wound with the palm of your hand and support your child in a semi-upright position. Reassure your child.

**2** With your child supported, cover the wound with a sterile dressing or clean pad and tape it in place on three sides, *far left*. Cover the pad with cling film to seal it; again secure tape on only three sides, *left*.

**3** Incline your child towards his injured side, supported with cushions. This helps support his chest.

☎ **CALL AN AMBULANCE**

>> **see also**
● Bleeding, *p.44*
● Shock, *p.30*
● Unconscious child, *pp.22–29*

# Abdominal wound

A child with an abdominal wound is likely to develop the signs of shock. There is high risk of internal as well as external bleeding.

**! IMPORTANT**

● **Monitor** your child for signs of shock.

● **If** your child loses consciousness, open her airway and check breathing. If breathing, place her in the recovery position, supporting her abdomen while you turn her. If she is not breathing, begin rescue breaths and chest compressions.

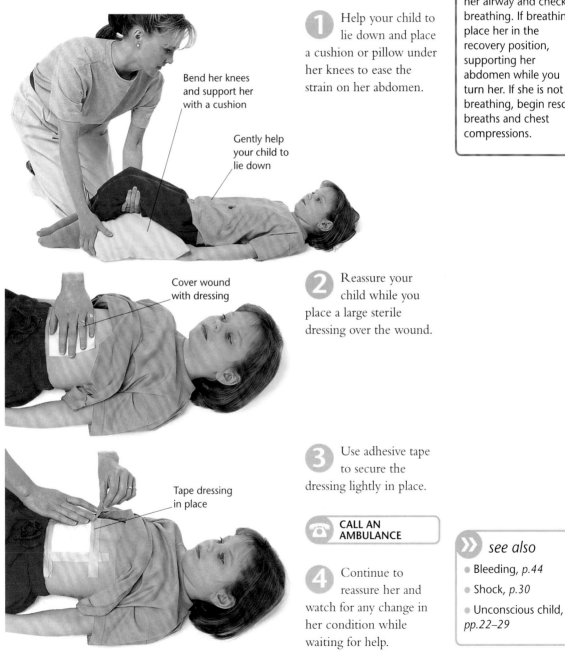

Bend her knees and support her with a cushion

Gently help your child to lie down

**1** Help your child to lie down and place a cushion or pillow under her knees to ease the strain on her abdomen.

Cover wound with dressing

**2** Reassure your child while you place a large sterile dressing over the wound.

Tape dressing in place

**3** Use adhesive tape to secure the dressing lightly in place.

☎ **CALL AN AMBULANCE**

**4** Continue to reassure her and watch for any change in her condition while waiting for help.

**» see also**

● Bleeding, *p.44*

● Shock, *p.30*

● Unconscious child, *pp.22–29*

# Burns and scalds

You must seek medical advice for all burns on children. A child with a large burn must be taken to hospital. It is very important to cool the burn as quickly as possible to minimise damage.

## Burns to the mouth and throat

Burns in this area are very serious as they cause swelling and inflammation of the air passages, giving a serious risk of suffocation. Act quickly. If necessary, loosen clothing from around her neck. If your child develops breathing difficulties, open her airway and check breathing. If she is not breathing begin rescue breaths and chest compressions. CALL AN AMBULANCE.

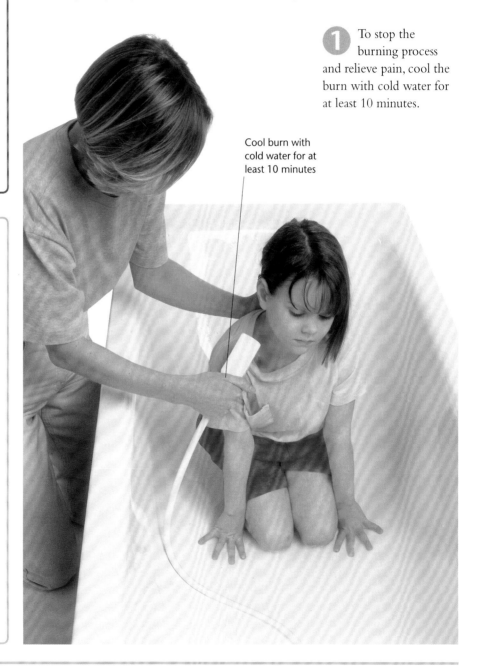

**1** To stop the burning process and relieve pain, cool the burn with cold water for at least 10 minutes.

Cool burn with cold water for at least 10 minutes

Remove cooled clothing and continue cooling injury

**2** Once cooled, remove clothing from the burned area and, if the pain persists, cool again. Cut around any material that is sticking to the skin. Remove jewellery and all restrictive clothing from around the burn (for example, belts or watches) before any swelling occurs.

### ⚠ IMPORTANT

● **Never** put lotions, fat, or ointment on a burn or scald.

● **If** the burn covers a large part of the child, CALL AN AMBULANCE.

● **Do not** give your child anything to eat or drink and watch for signs of shock.

● **If** child loses consciousness, open airway and check breathing. If breathing, place in the recovery position; if not breathing, begin rescue breaths and chest compressions. CALL AN AMBULANCE.

Cover burn loosely

**3** Cover the burn with cling film, a plastic bag, a clean sheet or pillow case. The dressing does not need to be secured. Keep your child warm to prevent hypothermia.

▶ **TAKE YOUR CHILD TO HOSPITAL**

### ⟫ see also

● Fire, *p.11*

● Shock, *p.30*

● Unconscious baby, *pp.17–21*

● Unconscious child, *pp.22–29*

## Using cling film

Open the roll, and discard the first few centimetres. Lay a piece of cling film lengthways along the injury. Never wrap it around the limb as the tissues swell.

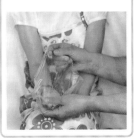

## ❗ IMPORTANT

● **Do not** touch your child until you are sure the electrical current is switched off.

● **Seek** medical advice for all burns to children.

● **If** no cold water is available, use another cool liquid such as milk.

● **If** child loses consciousness, open airway and check breathing. If breathing, place in the recovery position; if not breathing, begin rescue breaths and chest compressions. CALL AN AMBULANCE.

# Electrical burn

An electric shock from a low-voltage source can result in burns. These may occur at both the point of entry and the point of exit of the current.

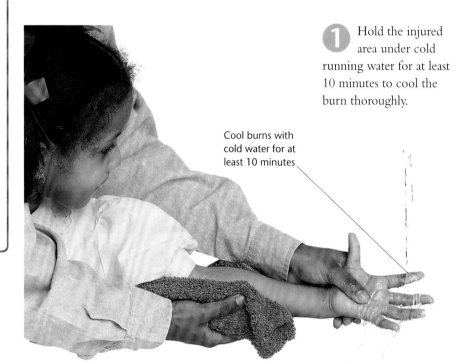

**1** Hold the injured area under cold running water for at least 10 minutes to cool the burn thoroughly.

Cool burns with cold water for at least 10 minutes

Cover burns on a hand with clean plastic bag

**2** Protect the burn by loosely covering it with cling film, a clean plastic bag, or clean material such as a pillow case.

## ≫ see also

● Electrical injury, *p.12*

● Unconscious baby, *pp.17–21*

● Unconscious child, *p.22–29*

▶ **TAKE YOUR CHILD TO HOSPITAL**

# Chemical burn to skin

Chemical burns can be caused by household agents such as oven cleaner or paint stripper. These burns are serious and there will be: fierce, stinging pain; redness or staining, followed by blistering and peeling of skin.

! **IMPORTANT**

● **Note** the name of the substance that caused the burn and give the information to the hospital staff.

● **Always** wear protective gloves when treating your child, and beware of chemical fumes.

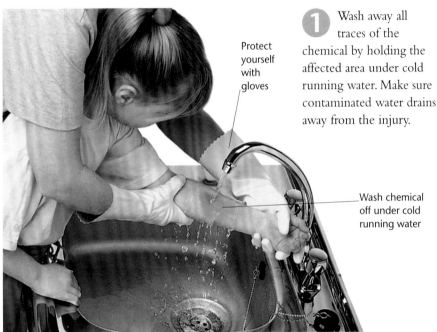

Protect yourself with gloves

Wash chemical off under cold running water

**1** Wash away all traces of the chemical by holding the affected area under cold running water. Make sure contaminated water drains away from the injury.

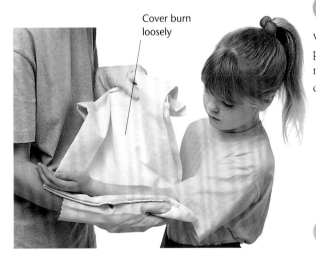

Cover burn loosely

**2** Protect the burn by loosely covering it with cling film, a clean plastic bag, or clean material such as a pillow case.

**TAKE YOUR CHILD TO HOSPITAL**

» *see also*

● Chemical burn to eye, *p.62*

● Fume inhalation, *p.41*

● Swallowed chemicals, *p.63*

> ! **IMPORTANT**
> * **Do not** let your child touch his eye. The eye will be shut in spasm and pain, so gently pull the eyelids open.

# Chemical burn to eye

Splashes of chemicals in the eye can cause scarring or even blindness. Your child may have a chemical burn if he complains of fierce pain in the eye; he has difficulty opening the affected eye; the surface of the eye is watery; there is redness and swelling in and around the eye.

## Using a jug of water

If you can't hold your child under a tap, you may find it easier to use a jug to pour water over the affected eye. Get a helper to support the child with her head tilted down and to one side. Avoid splashing the "good" eye with the contaminated water.

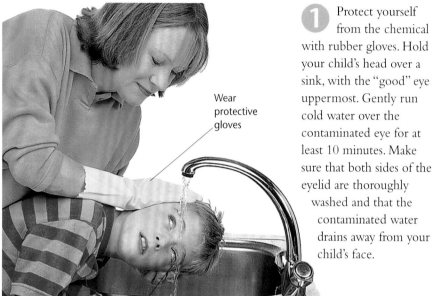

Wear protective gloves

Rinse eye with cold water for 10 minutes

Cover eye with clean pad

**1** Protect yourself from the chemical with rubber gloves. Hold your child's head over a sink, with the "good" eye uppermost. Gently run cold water over the contaminated eye for at least 10 minutes. Make sure that both sides of the eyelid are thoroughly washed and that the contaminated water drains away from your child's face.

**2** Once the injured eye is thoroughly washed, cover it with a large sterile dressing. Hold the dressing in place until you get medical aid.

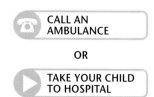

☎ **CALL AN AMBULANCE**

**OR**

▶ **TAKE YOUR CHILD TO HOSPITAL**

# Swallowed chemicals

If you think your child has swallowed a poison, try to find out what, when, and how much she has taken. Be aware too that some chemicals also give off dangerous fumes.

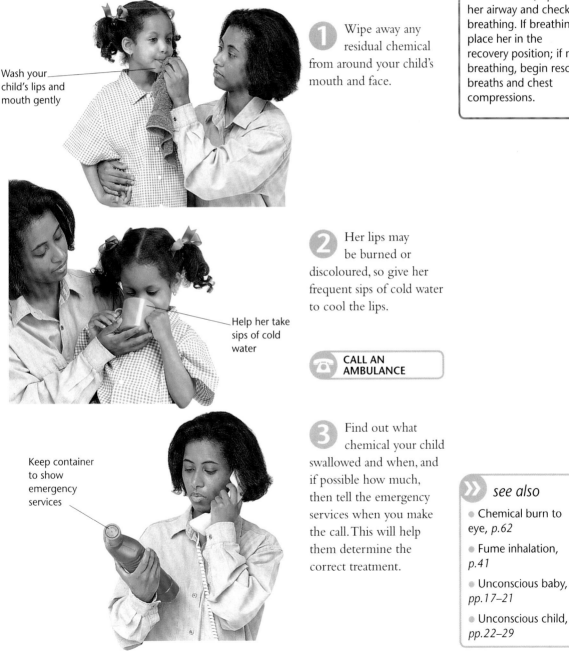

Wash your child's lips and mouth gently

**1** Wipe away any residual chemical from around your child's mouth and face.

**2** Her lips may be burned or discoloured, so give her frequent sips of cold water to cool the lips.

Help her take sips of cold water

**☎ CALL AN AMBULANCE**

Keep container to show emergency services

**3** Find out what chemical your child swallowed and when, and if possible how much, then tell the emergency services when you make the call. This will help them determine the correct treatment.

**》 see also**

● Chemical burn to eye, *p.62*

● Fume inhalation, *p.41*

● Unconscious baby, *pp.17–21*

● Unconscious child, *pp.22–29*

## ! IMPORTANT

● **Do not** make your child sick as it can cause further harm. If he is sick, give a sample to ambulance personnel.

● **Even** a small amount of alcohol may harm a young child.

● **If** your child is drowsy or loses consciousness, open airway and check breathing. If breathing, place him in the recovery position; if not breathing, begin rescue breaths and chest compressions.

## 》 see also

● Unconscious baby, pp.17–21

● Unconscious child, p.22–29

# Drug or alcohol poisoning

If your child has taken medication the container may be nearby. If he drank alcohol there may be a smell of alcohol and he may be staggering and be sick. He may also have: a flushed and moist face; slurred speech; deep noisy breathing; a bounding pulse.

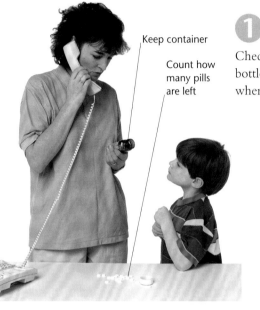

Keep container

Count how many pills are left

**1** Try to find out what he has taken, when, and how much. Check the label on the medicine bottle and tell ambulance control when you ring.

> ☎ **CALL AN AMBULANCE**

**2** If he drank alcohol, let your child rest where you can watch him while waiting for the ambulance. Give him a bowl in case he is sick. If he falls asleep, try to wake him to make sure he can be easily roused.

## ! IMPORTANT

● **Do not** make your child sick. This can cause further harm. If he is sick, keep a sample.

# Plant poisoning

Many plants are poisonous in large quantities. Small pieces or one or two berries are unlikely to be fatal but can cause stomach upset.

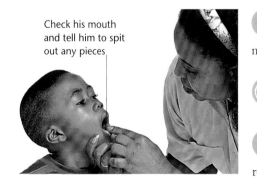

Check his mouth and tell him to spit out any pieces

**1** Try to find out what your child ate, when, and how much – keep a sample.

> ☎ **SEEK MEDICAL ADVICE**
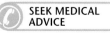

**2** Look inside your child's mouth. Pick out any remaining pieces of plant or berries.

# Scalp wound

This type of wound can bleed profusely. If the wound was caused by a blow to the child's head, watch for any change in her condition, especially her level of consciousness, while waiting for the ambulance.

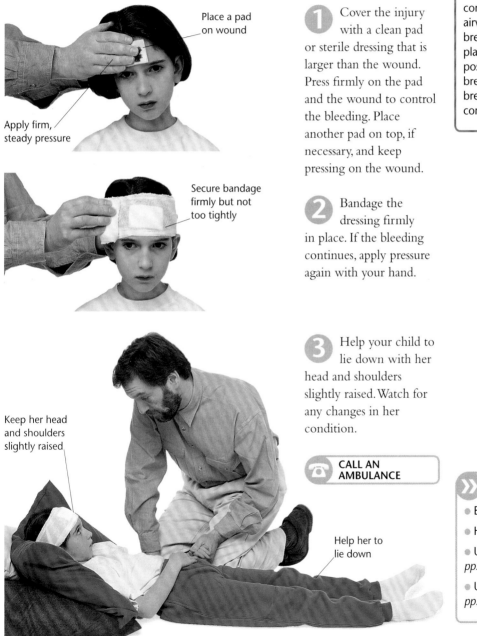

Place a pad on wound

Apply firm, steady pressure

Secure bandage firmly but not too tightly

Keep her head and shoulders slightly raised

Help her to lie down

**1** Cover the injury with a clean pad or sterile dressing that is larger than the wound. Press firmly on the pad and the wound to control the bleeding. Place another pad on top, if necessary, and keep pressing on the wound.

**2** Bandage the dressing firmly in place. If the bleeding continues, apply pressure again with your hand.

**3** Help your child to lie down with her head and shoulders slightly raised. Watch for any changes in her condition.

☎ **CALL AN AMBULANCE**

**❯❯** *see also*
● Bleeding, *p.44*
● Head injury, *p.66*
● Unconscious baby, *pp.17–21*
● Unconscious child, *pp.22–29*

**❗ IMPORTANT**
● **If** blood continues to seep through the two dressings, remove both pads and apply a new dressing.

● **If** your child loses consciousness, open her airway and check breathing. If breathing, place in the recovery position; if not breathing, begin rescue breaths and chest compressions.

## Skull fracture

Fractures of the skull are very serious injuries. Skull fracture can result in bleeding within the brain, which causes compression. Suspect skull fracture if there is: a wound on your child's head; a soft area on the scalp; consciousness is impaired; clear fluid coming from the nose or ear; blood showing on the white of the eye; or, distortion of the face or head. CALL AN AMBULANCE.

# Head injury

If your child has a minor bump to the head, he may simply have a small bruise with no other sign of injury. With concussion the child's brain is "shaken" by the blow; he may be dazed or temporarily unconscious (about 20 seconds), but recovers completely. He may have a headache, feel dizzy, complain of nausea, and may not remember what happened.

With compression, blood accumulates within the skull, pressing on the brain. The child may seem unaffected at first, however, hours (or days) later he deteriorates. He may be disorientated, drowsy, and confused. He may have: a severe headache; a fever; weakness or paralysis down one side; and unequal pupils. Eventually he will be unconscious with a strong, slow pulse, and noisy breathing that becomes very slow.

**1** If the child is dazed, help him to lie down on the ground. Don't sit him on a chair as he may fall and hurt himself.

**2** If your child was "knocked out" even briefly,

**SEEK MEDICAL ADVICE**

**3** Make him rest and watch him closely. Reassure him and stay with him. If he does not recover completely within 30 minutes,

**CALL AN AMBULANCE**

Help him to lie down

# Checking a child's level of consciousness

Your child could be awake following an injury, fully unconscious and not respond to you at all, or somewhere between the two. He may deteriorate. It is important to assess his condition and monitor any changes so that you can tell the ambulance personnel or hospital staff.

- Is he alert? Does he respond normally when you talk to him?

- Does he answer simple questions or obey instructions?

- Is he completely unresponsive?

Note down any response, or change in response (with the time of the change).

Put a cold compress on injury and monitor condition

# If your child loses consciousness

Do not move your child as there could be an associated back or neck injury and moving her could result in damage to the brain or spinal cord.

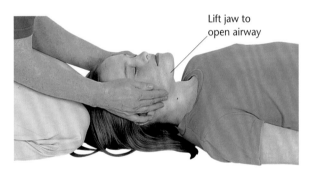

Lift jaw to open airway

1 Kneel behind her head and open her airway using the jaw thrust as follows. Place one hand on either side of her face, with your fingertips on the angles of her jaw. Gently lift the jaw to open the airway (don't tilt her head back).

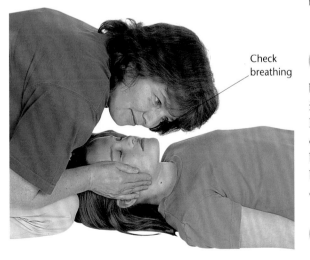

Check breathing

2 Check her breathing. If she is breathing, leave her as she is and continue to support her jaw to keep the airway open. If she is not breathing, begin rescue breaths and chest compressions.

**CALL AN AMBULANCE**

>> *see also*
- Cold compresses, *p.108*
- Spine injury, *pp.69–71*
- Scalp wound, *p.65*
- Unconscious baby, *pp.17–21*
- Unconscious child, *pp.22–29*

# Nose/cheekbone injury

The main risk with injuries to the nose or cheek is that the swelling can affect the air passages causing breathing problems. There may also be bleeding from the child's nose or mouth.

> **IMPORTANT**
> ● **If** pinching her nose hurts too much, simply ask her to sit forward over the bowl and give her a soft pad or towel to soak up the blood.

>> **see also**
● Nosebleed, *p.51*

● Unconscious baby, *pp.17–21*

● Unconscious child, *pp.22–29*

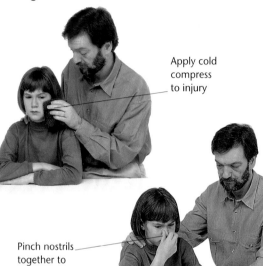

Apply cold compress to injury

Pinch nostrils together to stop bleeding

**1** Help your child to sit down and apply a cold compress to the injured area. This helps to reduce the swelling. Hold the compress in place for about 30 minutes.

**2** If your child's nose is bleeding heavily, ask her to sit with her head over a bowl and to pinch her nostrils together to help control it.

▶ **TAKE YOUR CHILD TO HOSPITAL**

# Jaw injury

If your child has a broken jaw it will be tender, swollen, and bruised. Her teeth may be out of line.

> **IMPORTANT**
> ● **If** your child loses consciousness, open airway and check her breathing. If not breathing, begin rescue breaths and chest compressions. CALL AN AMBULANCE.

>> **see also**
● Unconscious baby, *pp.17–21*

● Unconscious child, *p.22–29*

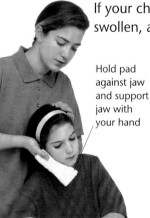

Hold pad against jaw and support jaw with your hand

**1** Help your child to sit down with head well forwards. Tell her not to swallow but to let any blood or saliva drain away.

**2** Make a soft pad and hold it firmly under her injured jaw. Do not bandage the pad in place in case she is sick. Continue to support the jaw on the way to the hospital.

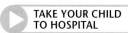

▶ **TAKE YOUR CHILD TO HOSPITAL**

# Spine injury

If a child lands on his neck or back in a fall or fell awkwardly and complains of back pain or tingling in any part of his body, suspect spine injury. Support him in the position you found him to minimise damage.

**!  IMPORTANT**

● **Do not** move the injured child unless his life is in danger.

● **If** you do have to move him, take care not to twist or bend the neck or spine, see page 71.

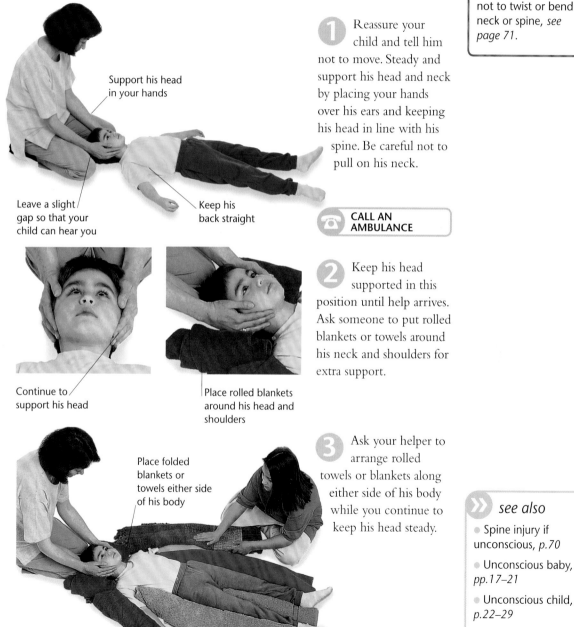

Support his head in your hands

Leave a slight gap so that your child can hear you

Keep his back straight

Continue to support his head

Place rolled blankets around his head and shoulders

Place folded blankets or towels either side of his body

**1** Reassure your child and tell him not to move. Steady and support his head and neck by placing your hands over his ears and keeping his head in line with his spine. Be careful not to pull on his neck.

☎ **CALL AN AMBULANCE**

**2** Keep his head supported in this position until help arrives. Ask someone to put rolled blankets or towels around his neck and shoulders for extra support.

**3** Ask your helper to arrange rolled towels or blankets along either side of his body while you continue to keep his head steady.

**» see also**

● Spine injury if unconscious, p.70

● Unconscious baby, pp.17–21

● Unconscious child, p.22–29

> ! **IMPORTANT**
> • **Do not** move him unless his life is in immediate danger.
> • **If** you are alone and need to leave your child to call an ambulance, and your child remains unconscious, place him in the recovery position before you leave him.

# Spine injury if unconscious

If your child is unconscious following a fall on to his back, you should follow the usual steps to treat unconsciousness, but you need to adapt how you open his airway to prevent movement of the back or neck.

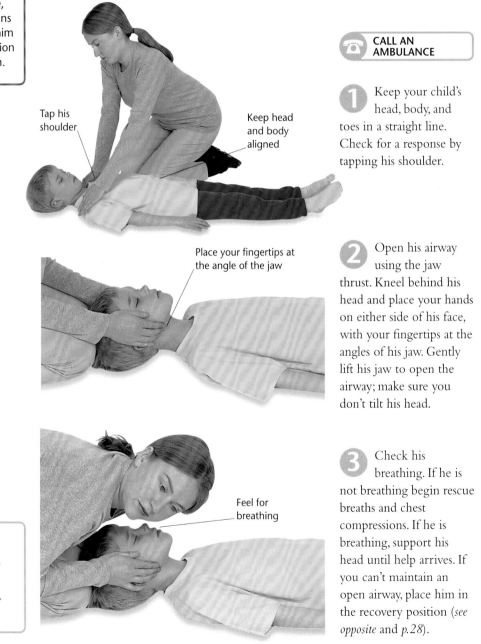

Tap his shoulder

Keep head and body aligned

Place your fingertips at the angle of the jaw

Feel for breathing

☎ CALL AN AMBULANCE

**1** Keep your child's head, body, and toes in a straight line. Check for a response by tapping his shoulder.

**2** Open his airway using the jaw thrust. Kneel behind his head and place your hands on either side of his face, with your fingertips at the angles of his jaw. Gently lift his jaw to open the airway; make sure you don't tilt his head.

**3** Check his breathing. If he is not breathing begin rescue breaths and chest compressions. If he is breathing, support his head until help arrives. If you can't maintain an open airway, place him in the recovery position (*see opposite* and *p.28*).

>> **see also**
• Unconscious baby, *pp.17–21*
• Unconscious child, *p.22–29*

# If you have one helper

If your child is breathing and you cannot maintain an open airway using the jaw thrust, for example, if he vomits, place him in the recovery position.

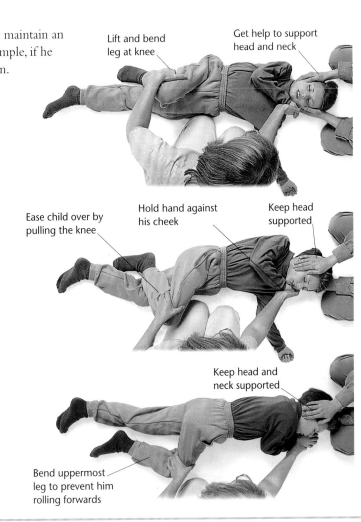

Lift and bend leg at knee

Get help to support head and neck

**1** Ask your helper to support your child's head with her hands. Bring his furthest arm across his chest and hold his hand against his cheek. Pull up the knee of the furthest leg to bend the leg.

Ease child over by pulling the knee

Hold hand against his cheek

Keep head supported

**2** Still holding the hand against his cheek, pull your child's knee towards you and roll him onto his side. You and the helper should keep his head and body aligned at all times.

Keep head and neck supported

**3** With your child on his side, maintain an open airway and support him in this position until help arrives. Monitor his breathing and pulse. If he stops breathing you will need to roll him onto his back to begin rescue breaths and chest compressions without delay.

Bend uppermost leg to prevent him rolling forwards

# For two or more helpers

If you have two or more adult helpers, use the "log-roll" technique to turn a child. It is vital to keep his head, body, and feet in a straight line. While one adult holds the child's head, two others should gently straighten the limbs and roll the child over in one synchronised movement.

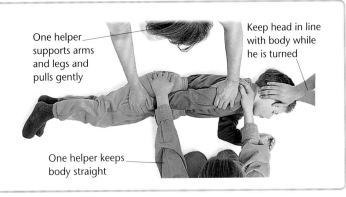

One helper supports arms and legs and pulls gently

Keep head in line with body while he is turned

One helper keeps body straight

**!  IMPORTANT**

● **Do** not bandage if it causes pain.

● **If** there is bleeding but no obvious wound, treat for shock.

● **If** your child is very uncomfortable, placing cushions under the knees may help alleviate the pain.

**»  see also**

● Shock, *p.30*

# Pelvic injury

If your child has a broken pelvis she will be unable to stand, with pain around the hip and groin, and possible bleeding from the urinary orifice.

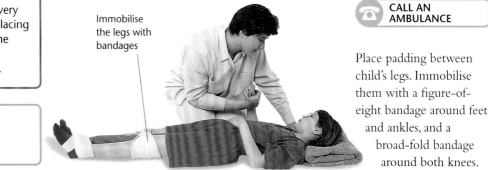

Immobilise the legs with bandages

**☎  CALL AN AMBULANCE**

Place padding between child's legs. Immobilise them with a figure-of-eight bandage around feet and ankles, and a broad-fold bandage around both knees.

**!  IMPORTANT**

● **If** there is a wound treat bleeding and cover it with a dressing.

# Leg injury

Suspect a break if your child is in severe pain. He needs an X-ray or scan to confirm whether or not a bone is broken. Keep him as still as possible to prevent broken bone ends causing further internal injury.

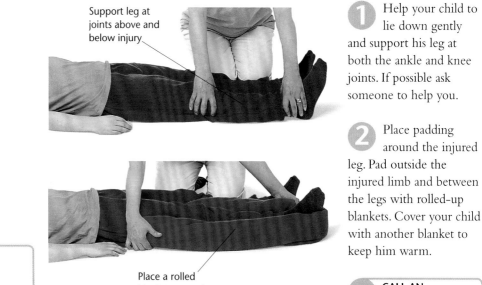

Support leg at joints above and below injury

**1** Help your child to lie down gently and support his leg at both the ankle and knee joints. If possible ask someone to help you.

**2** Place padding around the injured leg. Pad outside the injured limb and between the legs with rolled-up blankets. Cover your child with another blanket to keep him warm.

Place a rolled blanket around his leg

**»  see also**

● Bleeding, *p.44*

**☎  CALL AN AMBULANCE**

# How to splint an injured leg

If you are going to have to wait for help, for example if in a remote area, splint the injured leg for extra support.

**1** Gently pad between the thighs, knees, and ankles using rolled-up towels or small blankets. Carefully bring the uninjured leg alongside the broken limb.

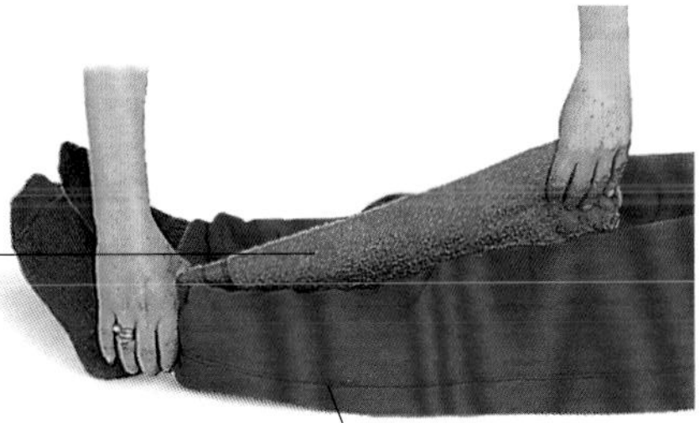

Place plenty of soft padding between the legs

Support injured leg

**2** Tie a narrow-fold figure-of-eight bandage around the feet and ankles to immobilise the leg.

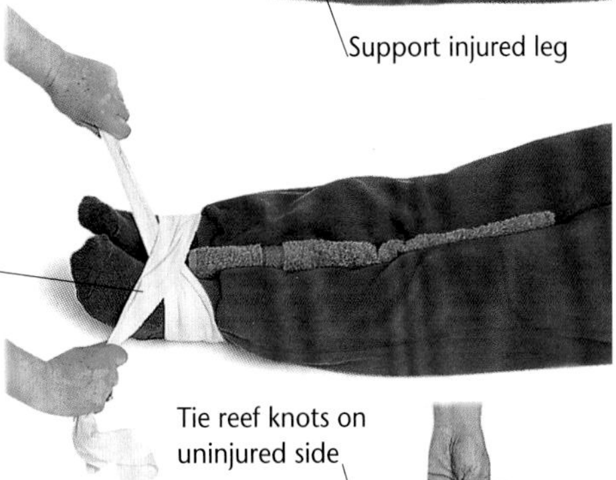

Tie narrow-fold bandage in figure-of-eight at ankles and feet

**3** Tie broad-fold bandages around the knee, and above as well as below the injury if there is room.

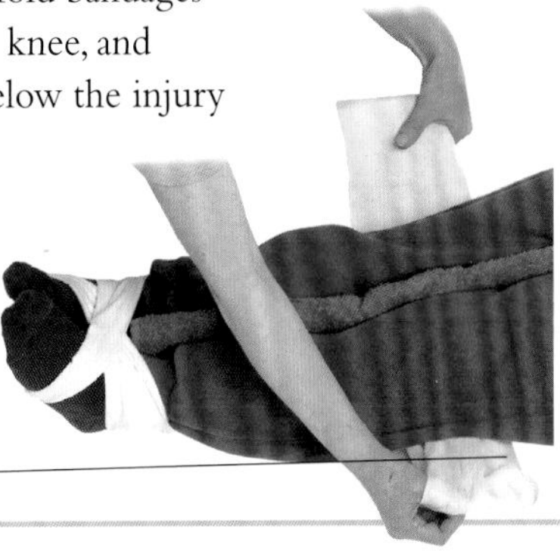

Tie reef knots on uninjured side

Tie broad-fold bandages at knees and above and below injury

Slide broad-fold under knee and tie ends together

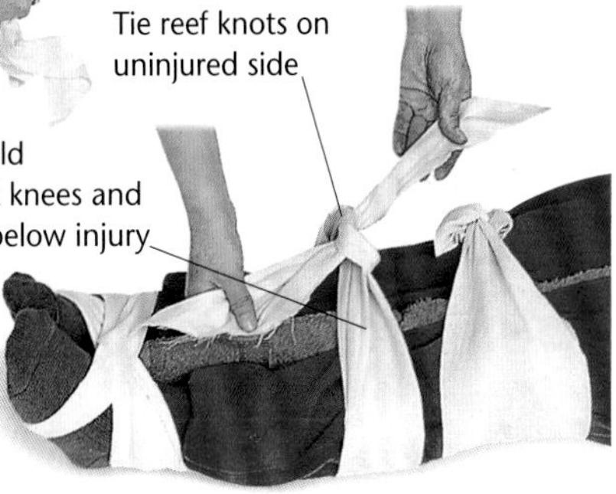

# Making broad-fold and narrow-fold bandages

**1** 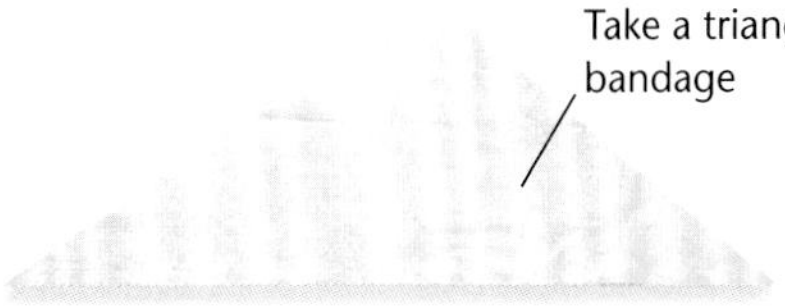 Take a triangular bandage

**2** 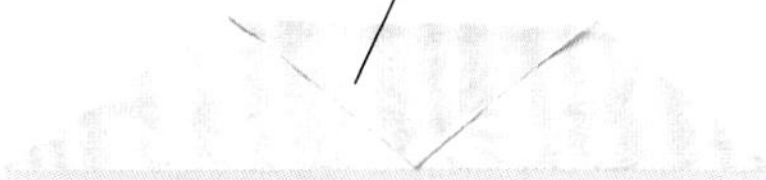 Fold top point over to touch the base

**3** Fold bandage in half to make a broad-fold bandage

Broad-fold Bandage

**4** Fold bandage in half again to make a narrow-fold bandage

Narrow-fold Bandage

# Knee injury

This type of injury can be very painful, and your child may not be able to move it. The area around the knee joint can swell very quickly.

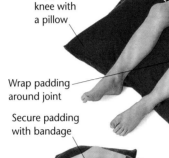

Support his knee with a pillow

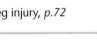

Wrap padding around joint

Secure padding with bandage

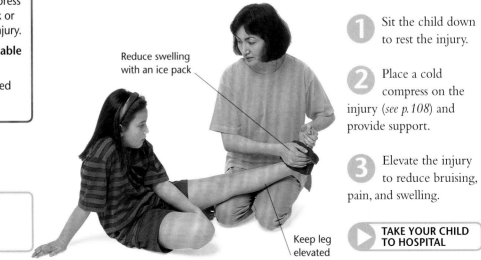

Keep him comfortable

**1** Help your child to lie down, then slide a pillow under his legs and place a cold compress on the knee. Provide comfortable support. Wrap a thick layer of soft padding around the knee.

**2** Secure the padding with a bandage. Reassure the child.

>> **CALL AN AMBULANCE**

>> *see also*
● Leg injury, *p.72*

---

# Foot injury

Your child's foot may be bruised, swollen, and stiff and she may not be able to stand. If caused by crushing, one or more bones may be broken.

Reduce swelling with an ice pack

**1** Sit the child down to rest the injury.

**2** Place a cold compress on the injury (*see p.108*) and provide support.

**3** Elevate the injury to reduce bruising, pain, and swelling.

Keep leg elevated

>> **TAKE YOUR CHILD TO HOSPITAL**

>> *see also*
● Leg injury, *p.72*

# Ankle injury

The most common injury is a sprain. Suspect a sprain if your child can't take her full weight on her foot after a fall, or she has twisted, or wrenched, her ankle. She may need an X-ray or scan.

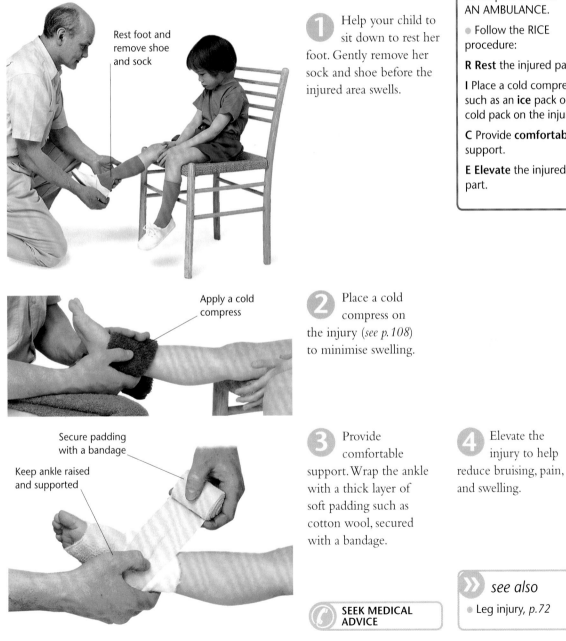

Rest foot and remove shoe and sock

Apply a cold compress

Secure padding with a bandage

Keep ankle raised and supported

**1** Help your child to sit down to rest her foot. Gently remove her sock and shoe before the injured area swells.

**2** Place a cold compress on the injury (*see p.108*) to minimise swelling.

**3** Provide comfortable support. Wrap the ankle with a thick layer of soft padding such as cotton wool, secured with a bandage.

**4** Elevate the injury to help reduce bruising, pain, and swelling.

**SEEK MEDICAL ADVICE**

**»** *see also*
● Leg injury, *p.72*

# Collar bone injury

A collar bone may be broken by indirect force, for example, if a child falls onto her outstretched hand, or by a blow to her shoulder. There will be tenderness in your child's shoulder and arm – increased by attempts to move it – and her head will be turned and inclined to the injured side.

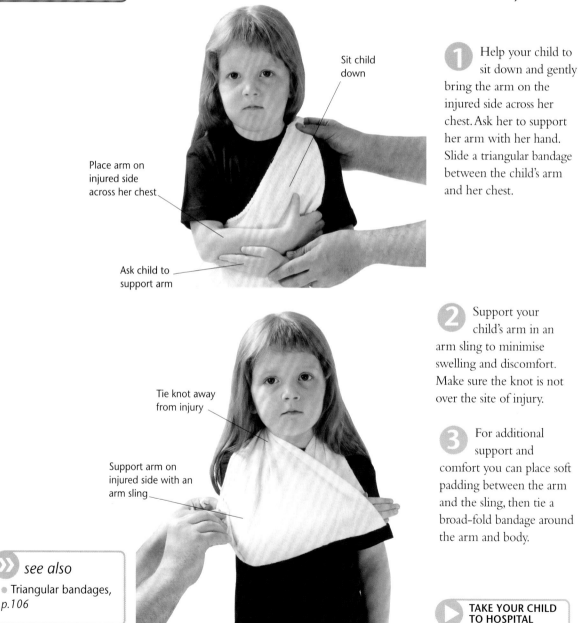

Sit child down

Place arm on injured side across her chest

Ask child to support arm

Tie knot away from injury

Support arm on injured side with an arm sling

**1** Help your child to sit down and gently bring the arm on the injured side across her chest. Ask her to support her arm with her hand. Slide a triangular bandage between the child's arm and her chest.

**2** Support your child's arm in an arm sling to minimise swelling and discomfort. Make sure the knot is not over the site of injury.

**3** For additional support and comfort you can place soft padding between the arm and the sling, then tie a broad-fold bandage around the arm and body.

**≫ see also**

● Triangular bandages, p.106

▶ **TAKE YOUR CHILD TO HOSPITAL**

# Rib injury

A child may have a broken rib following a blow to her chest, a heavy fall, or having been crushed. Symptoms include: sharp pain at the fracture site; and pain on breathing.

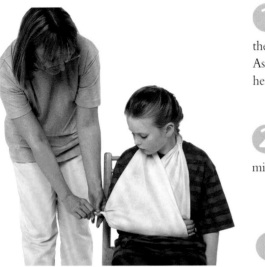

**1** Help your child to sit down and gently bring the arm on the injured side across her chest. Ask her to support her arm with her hand.

**2** Support your child's arm in an arm sling to minimise discomfort.

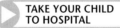
▶ TAKE YOUR CHILD TO HOSPITAL

**❗ IMPORTANT**

● **If** your child loses consciousness or develops breathing difficulties, open airway and check breathing. If breathing place her in the recovery position leaning on the injured side; if not breathing, begin rescue breaths and chest compressions.

**》 see also**

● Chest wound, *p.56*
● Internal bleeding, *p.55*
● Shock, *p.30*
● Triangular bandages, *p.106*
● Unconscious child, *pp.22–29*

## For severe rib injury

Suspect internal injury if you see signs of internal bleeding or an wound. If there is a wound, or several ribs are injured support the chest wall to safeguard breathing.

**1** Support your child in a semi-upright position leaning towards his injured side. Seal any chest wound: place a sterile pad over the wound, cover this with kitchen film secured on three sides with tape.

**2** Place the arm on the injured side across your child's chest for extra support. Secure it with an elevation sling. Keep him as comfortable as possible while you wait for the ambulance.

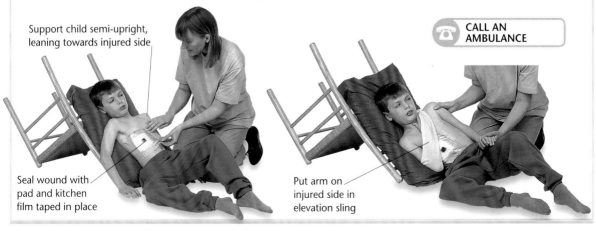

Support child semi-upright, leaning towards injured side

Seal wound with pad and kitchen film taped in place

☎ CALL AN AMBULANCE

Put arm on injured side in elevation sling

**! IMPORTANT**

● **If** the child cannot bend his arm treat as for elbow injury below. CALL AN AMBULANCE.

# Arm injury

The treatment below is suitable for injuries to the upper arm, forearm, and wrist. Move the injured arm as little as possible.

Place padding around injury

**1** Help your child to sit down and, if possible, get him to support his injured arm with his other hand. Place a soft pad between his arm and his chest to protect and cushion the injured limb.

Support arm in a sling

**2** Immobilise the injured arm by supporting it in an arm sling. Secure the sling with a knot.

Ask him to support injury until sling is secure

**》》 see also**

● Triangular bandages, p.106

**▶ TAKE YOUR CHILD TO HOSPITAL**

---

**! IMPORTANT**

● **Do not** attempt to straighten or bend your child's elbow.

# Elbow injury

Elbow injuries need early treatment in hospital. Suspect elbow injury if your child is unable to bend his arm; pain is increased by any attempts at movement; there is swelling or bruising around the elbow.

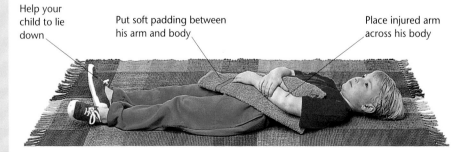

Help your child to lie down

Put soft padding between his arm and body

Place injured arm across his body

Help your child to lie down and place his arm in the most comfortable position. Support it with cushions if necessary.

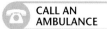

**☎ CALL AN AMBULANCE**

# Hand injury

This type of injury can be very painful. There may be several broken bones, and often a joint is dislocated. If your child's hand was crushed there may also be an open wound. Your child will need an X-ray or scan.

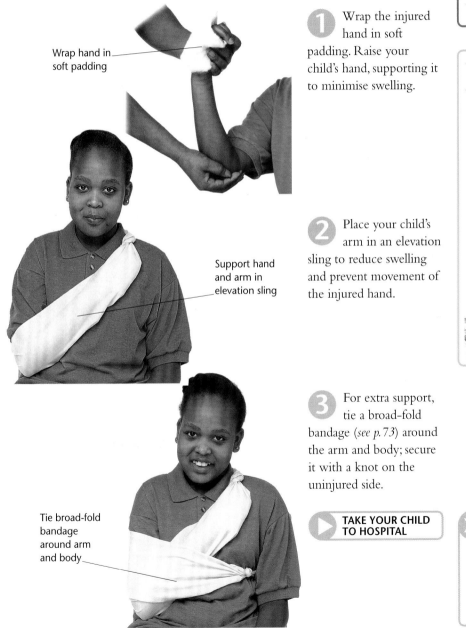

Wrap hand in soft padding

Support hand and arm in elevation sling

Tie broad-fold bandage around arm and body

**1** Wrap the injured hand in soft padding. Raise your child's hand, supporting it to minimise swelling.

**2** Place your child's arm in an elevation sling to reduce swelling and prevent movement of the injured hand.

**3** For extra support, tie a broad-fold bandage (*see p. 73*) around the arm and body; secure it with a knot on the uninjured side.

▶ **TAKE YOUR CHILD TO HOSPITAL**

## ! IMPORTANT

● **If** there is a wound, control the bleeding by raising the hand and gently press a clean dressing or pad over the site of the wound.

## Trapped fingers

Hold the fingers under cold running water for a few minutes to relieve the pain and minimise swelling. If the fingers still hurt, apply a cold compress (*see p. 108*).

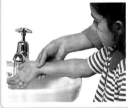

## ›› see also

● Bleeding, *p.44*

● Crush injury, *p.55*

● Triangular bandages, *p.106*

# Bruises and swellings

After a fall or bump, bruising and swelling may develop rapidly. Resting, cooling, and raising the injury will minimise discomfort.

## Cold compresses

Applying a cold compress helps minimise swelling and discomfort by reducing blood flow to the area. Make one by filling a plastic bag two-thirds full of ice or use a bag of frozen fruit or vegetables. Wrap the bag in a tea towel. A cloth wrung out in cold water can also be used (*see p.108*).

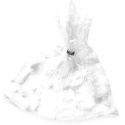

Leave a compress in place on an injury for about 30 minutes, ideally uncovered.

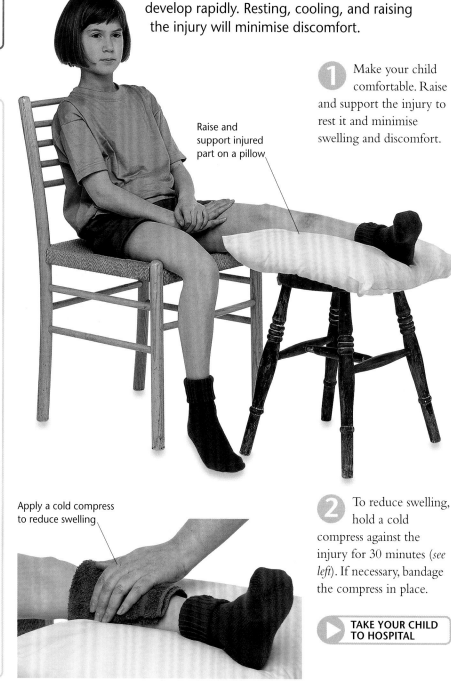

Raise and support injured part on a pillow

1 Make your child comfortable. Raise and support the injury to rest it and minimise swelling and discomfort.

Apply a cold compress to reduce swelling

2 To reduce swelling, hold a cold compress against the injury for 30 minutes (*see left*). If necessary, bandage the compress in place.

▶ **TAKE YOUR CHILD TO HOSPITAL**

# Splinter

There is always a risk of infection with splinters. They are often dirty and the bacteria can be carried deep into the skin. Children are most likely to get splinters in their hands and knees as they crawl on the floor.

**!**  **IMPORTANT**

- **If** your child is not immunised against tetanus infection, SEEK MEDICAL ADVICE.

- **Do not** poke at the area with a needle to remove the splinter.

- **If** you cannot remove the splinter, or if it breaks off, SEEK MEDICAL ADVICE.

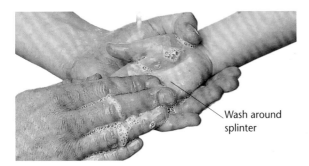

**1** Clean the area around the splinter thoroughly with soap and warm water.

Wash around splinter

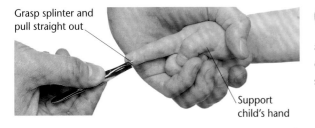

Grasp splinter and pull straight out

**2** Grasp the splinter as close to the skin as possible, and carefully draw it back out at the same angle it went in.

Support child's hand

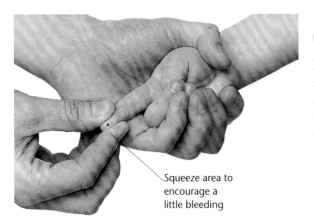

**3** Squeeze the wound to encourage a little bleeding that will flush out dirt. Wash the area again, pat it dry thoroughly, and cover with a plaster.

Squeeze area to encourage a little bleeding

**»** *see also*
- Infected wound, *p.48*

! **IMPORTANT**

● **Do not** touch, or attempt to remove, any foreign object that is sticking to, or embedded in, the eye. TAKE YOUR CHILD TO HOSPITAL.

● **If** eye is still red or sore after the object has been removed, TAKE HER TO HOSPITAL.

## For an object that cannot be removed

Tell your child to keep his eyes still, and cover his eye with a sterile dressing. Reassure him. TAKE HIM TO HOSPITAL.

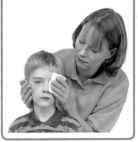

» *see also*
● Eye wound, *p.50*

# Object in eye

Tiny hairs or specks of dust on the surface of the eye can be very uncomfortable for a child. However, anything on the surface can generally be washed off easily; try to prevent your child rubbing her eye.

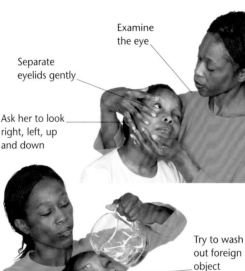

Examine the eye

Separate eyelids gently

Ask her to look right, left, up and down

Try to wash out foreign object

Use a bowl to catch water

Lift upper eyelid over lower lid

**1** Help your child to sit down, facing the light. Separate the eyelids of the affected eye. Ask her to look right, left, up, and down. Examine her eye thoroughly.

**2** If you can see the foreign object on the surface of the eye, try to wash it off using a jug of clean water. Tilt her head and aim for the inner corner so that water will wash over her eye. Or, try lifting it off with a damp swab or the corner of a handkerchief.

**3** If an object is under the eyelid, you can ask an older child to clear it by lifting the upper eyelid over the lower one. You will need to do this for a younger child; if necessary, wrap her in a towel first to stop her grabbing your arms.

# Object in ear

Children often push things into their ears. A hard object may become stuck, which can cause pain and temporary deafness; it may even damage the child's ear drum.

Find out what is in the ear but don't try to remove it

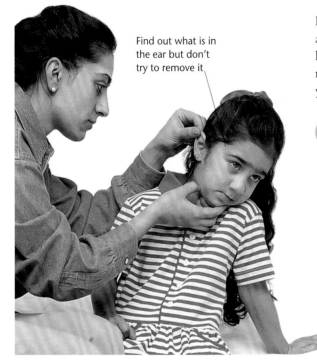

Reassure your child and ask her what she put into her ear. Don't try to remove the object, even if you can see it.

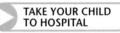

▶ **TAKE YOUR CHILD TO HOSPITAL**

## If there is an insect in the ear

If an insect flies or crawls into your child's ear she may be very alarmed.

**1** Help her to sit her down. Support her head with the affected ear uppermost.

**2** Gently flood the ear with tepid water so that the insect floats out.

# Object in nose

If your child has something stuck in his nose his breathing may be difficult or noisy and his nose may be swollen. Smelly or blood-stained discharge from the nose indicates an object has been present for a while.

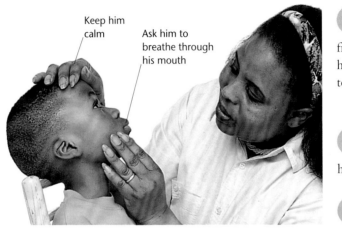

Keep him calm

Ask him to breathe through his mouth

**1** Reassure your child and try to find out what he put in his nose. Tell him not to touch it.

**2** Tell your child to breathe through his mouth.

▶ **TAKE YOUR CHILD TO HOSPITAL**

# Swallowed object

Young children often put small objects in their mouths and may swallow them. Most objects will pass straight through the digestive system. Small button batteries are dangerous as they contain corrosive chemicals.

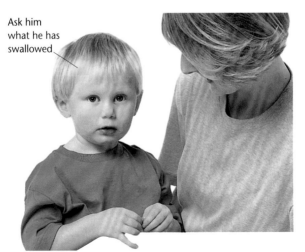

Ask him what he has swallowed

**1** Reassure your child. Try to find out what he child has swallowed.

**2** If the object is small and smooth like a pebble or a coin, there is little danger.

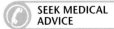
📞 **SEEK MEDICAL ADVICE**

# Animal and human bites

The main risk with any bite is infection; sharp pointed teeth can carry germs deep into the skin. Severe wounds with torn edges may need stitches. There is a risk of rabies from animals from outside the UK.

**!** **IMPORTANT**

● **If** the bleeding is severe, treat your child for shock.

● **If** your child is bitten by an animal while you are abroad, you must take your child to hospital for advice about rabies.

● **Make** sure child's tetanus immunisation is up to date.

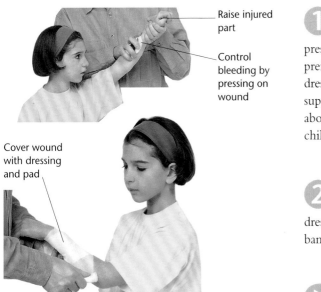

Raise injured part

Control bleeding by pressing on wound

Cover wound with dressing and pad

**1** If bleeding is severe, apply direct pressure over the wound, preferably over a clean dressing or pad. Raise and support the injured part above the level of your child's heart.

**2** Cover the wound with a sterile dressing or pad and bandage firmly in place.

**》** *see also*

● Bleeding, *p.44*

● Infected wound, *p.48*

● Shock, *p.30*

▶ **TAKE YOUR CHILD TO HOSPITAL**

## For a superficial animal bite

**1** Wash the wound thoroughly, using soap and warm water. Rinse the wound under running water for at least five minutes to wash away any dirt.

**2** Gently, but thoroughly, pat the wound dry with a clean pad or tissue. Cover it with a plaster or a small sterile dressing.

⟳ **SEEK MEDICAL ADVICE**

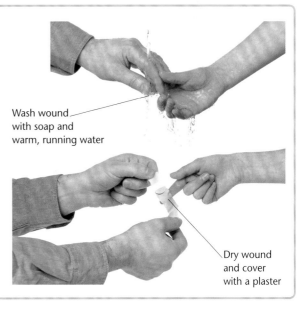

Wash wound with soap and warm, running water

Dry wound and cover with a plaster

**!  IMPORTANT**

● **If child collapses, she
may be allergic to the
sting. Treat for
anaphylactic shock.**

# Insect sting

Bee, wasp, or hornet stings can be very alarming for a child, but they are
rarely dangerous. Your child will experience a sharp pain followed by
soreness, red skin, and slight swelling around the site of the sting.

## If sting is in mouth

To reduce swelling, give
your child an ice cube
to suck or cold water
to drink. SEEK
MEDICAL ADVICE.
If breathing becomes
difficult, CALL AN
AMBULANCE.

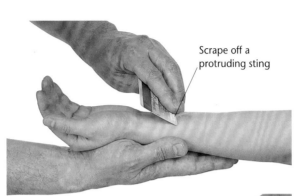

Scrape off a
protruding sting

Place a cold
compress over area

**1** If the sting is still in
the skin, brush or
scrape it off sideways with
your fingernail or a plastic
card. Do not try to
remove it with tweezers
as you will inject more
poison into your child.

**2** Cool the area with
a cold compress to
minimise the pain and
swelling. Leave the
compress in place for
about ten minutes, until
the pain is relieved. Rest
the injured part.

**»  see also**

● Anaphylactic shock,
*opposite*

---

**!  IMPORTANT**

● **If the rash is extensive,
SEEK MEDICAL ADVICE.**

# Nettle rash

If your child brushes against nettles he will have a blotchy, red, itchy rash
that may frighten him. Reassure him and soothe the rash.

Soothe rash by
dabbing with
calamine lotion

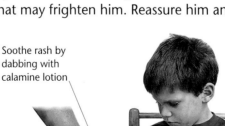

**1** To relieve the
itching, dab the
rash with cotton wool
soaked in calamine lotion.

**2** Alternatively, place
a cold compress
over the rash until the
pain is relieved, about 10
minutes.

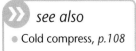

**»  see also**

● Cold compress, *p.108*

# Anaphylactic shock

This is a severe allergic reaction that may develop within a few minutes of the injection of a drug, an insect or marine creature sting, or ingestion of a food. It causes constriction of the air passages and swelling of the face and neck that can result in suffocation. Suspect anaphylactic shock if your child also develops red, itchy, blotchy skin, has difficulty breathing, abdominal pain, vomiting, and diarrhoea.

Support her in a position that helps her breathing

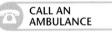 **CALL AN AMBULANCE**

**1** Help your child into the position that most relieves her breathing difficulty.

**2** Talk to her calmly and reassure her while you wait for the ambulance to arrive.

> **! IMPORTANT**
>
> ● **If** your child loses consciousness, open her airway and check breathing. If breathing, place in the recovery position; if not breathing, begin rescue breaths and chest compressions.
>
> ● **If** child has her own medication help her to use it or, give it to her yourself, *see below*.

》 *see also*
● Shock, *p.30*

---

## Administering an auto-injector

A child with a known allergy may have her own medication to take in case of an attack. This usually takes the form of an auto-injector of adrenaline prescribed for the child's own use.

**1** Hold the injector with your fingers and remove the safety cap.

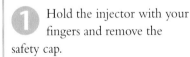
Tip

Safety cap

Inject medication into thigh muscle through her clothing

**2** Holding the injector with your fist, place the tip firmly against the child's thigh to release the medication. Rub the injection site.

**!** **IMPORTANT**

● **If** your child develops a severe allergic reaction, treat as for anaphylactic shock and CALL AN AMBULANCE.

● **If** the sting is caused by a tropical jellyfish, pour vinegar or sea water over injury and CALL AN AMBULANCE.

● **If** the skin is very red and painful, TAKE YOUR CHILD TO HOSPITAL.

# Jellyfish sting

Jellyfish venom is contained in stinging cells that stick to a child's skin. The sting is painful, but not usually serious. A similar reaction is produced by sea anemones and corals.

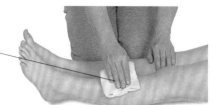

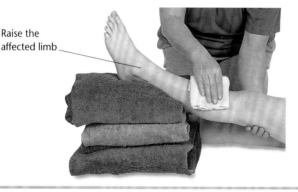

Cool the affected area with a compress

**1** Apply a cold compress against the skin. Leave the compress on the wound for about 10 minutes.

Raise the affected limb

**2** If possible, raise and support the affected part to reduce swelling.

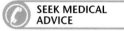

**SEEK MEDICAL ADVICE**

**»** *see also*

● Anaphylactic shock, *p.87*

● Cold compresses, *p.108*

---

**!** **IMPORTANT**

● **Make** sure the water is not too hot.

● **If** any spines remain embedded in the skin, or the foot starts to swell, TAKE YOUR CHILD TO THE HOSPITAL

# Weever fish sting

When trodden on, the spines from a weever fish can puncture the skin, causing painful swelling and soreness. The spines can also break off and become embedded in a child's foot.

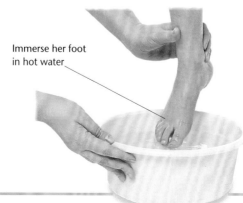

Immerse her foot in hot water

Immerse the injury in water as hot as your child can bear for at least 30 minutes. Top up as the water cools but be careful not to scald her.

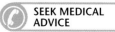

**SEEK MEDICAL ADVICE**

# Snake bite

If your child is bitten by a snake there will be two puncture marks. There may also be redness at the site and he may be feeling sick or vomiting, and be sweating. There may be disturbed vision and difficulty breathing.

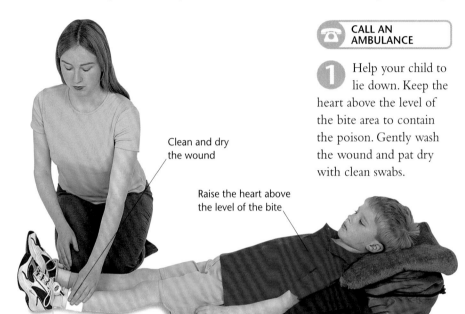

Clean and dry the wound

Raise the heart above the level of the bite

☎ **CALL AN AMBULANCE**

**1** Help your child to lie down. Keep the heart above the level of the bite area to contain the poison. Gently wash the wound and pat dry with clean swabs.

> **! IMPORTANT**
>
> ● **If** your child develops a severe allergic reaction, treat as for anaphylactic shock.
>
> ● **If** your child loses consciousness, open his airway and check breathing. If breathing, place in the recovery position; if not breathing, begin rescue breaths and chest compressions.
>
> ● **Do not** let your child walk about.
>
> ● **Do not** apply a tourniquet, cut out the wound, or try to suck out the venom.
>
> ● **If** possible give an accurate description of the snake to the emergency services to help them with treatment.

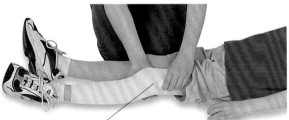

Apply roller bandage above bite

**2** Lightly compress the whole limb above the bite with a roller bandage. If the hand or foot begins to feel numb or cold, loosen the bandage slightly.

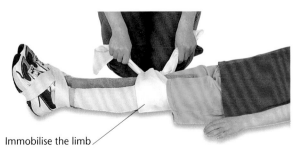

Immobilise the limb

**3** Immobilise the limb with folded triangular bandages and padding. Reassure your child and keep him still to stop the venom spreading through his body.

> **»» see also**
>
> ● Anaphylactic shock, *p.87*
> ● Triangular bandages, *p.106*
> ● Unconscious baby, *pp.17–21*
> ● Unconscious child, *p.22–29*

# Hypothermia

This develops if the body temperature falls. Deep hypothermia, where the body temperature falls very low, is extremely serious. An older child is most likely to develop it outside in poor weather conditions, or after falling into cold water. For babies, *see opposite*. Your child is suffering from hypothermia if she is shivering and has cold, pale, dry skin; she is listless or confused and is losing consciousness; and she has slow, shallow breathing and a weakening pulse.

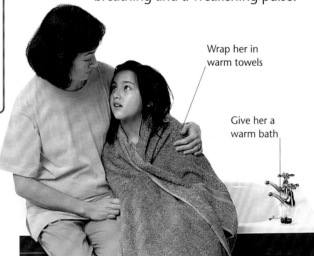

Wrap her in warm towels

Give her a warm bath

**1**  If your child is able to climb into a bath, give her a warm bath. When her skin colour has returned to normal, help her out, dry her quickly, and wrap her in warm towels or blankets. If she cannot climb into a bath go to step 2.

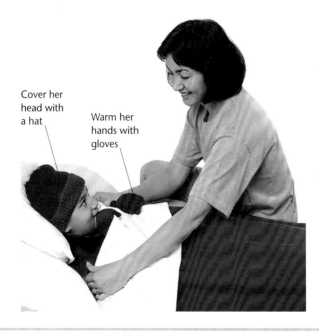

Cover her head with a hat

Warm her hands with gloves

**2**  Dress your child with warm clothes and put her to bed, covered with plenty of blankets. Cover her head with a hat and make sure that the room is warm. Stay with her.

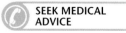
**SEEK MEDICAL ADVICE**

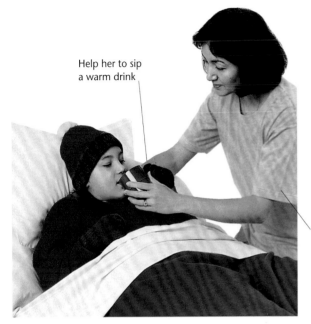

Help her to sip a warm drink

**3** Give your child a warm drink and some high-energy foods, such as chocolate. Do not leave her alone until you are sure that her colour and temperature have returned to normal.

Stay with her until colour and temperature have returned to normal

**see also**
● Unconscious baby, *pp.17–21*
● Unconscious child, *p.22–29*

## Hypothermia in babies

A baby's temperature regulation is not fully developed. He can lose body heat rapidly and develop hypothermia in a cold room. A hypothermic baby must be warmed gradually. Suspect hypothermia if your baby: is pink and healthy looking but skin feels cold; seems limp and unusually quiet; and he refuses to feed.

☎ **CALL AN AMBULANCE**

**1** Warm a baby gradually. Take him into a warm room. Wrap him in blankets.

**2** Put a hat on his head and cuddle him against your body so that he is warmed by your body heat.

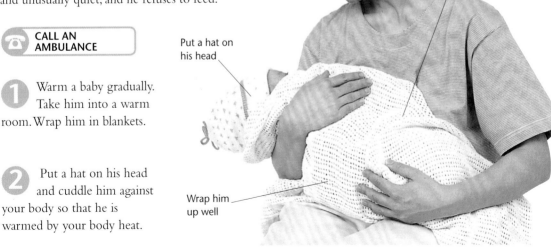

Cuddle him against your body

Put a hat on his head

Wrap him up well

# Frostbite

If children are exposed to extreme weather conditions, the tissues of the fingers and toes may freeze. Your child may have frostbite if she has pins and needles in her fingers or toes with numbness and hard, stiff skin that is turning white and waxy. Shelter your child before treating her.

## If recovery is slow or skin broken

If there are any open wounds, the frozen skin is broken, or the colour does not return rapidly, cover the area with a soft gauze dressing and bandage it lightly in place. TAKE YOUR CHILD TO THE HOSPITAL.

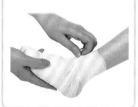

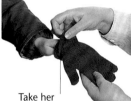

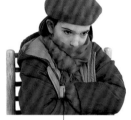

Take her gloves off very carefully

Warm hands with her own body heat, under armpits

**1** Take your child into a warm shelter before you start treatment. Help her to sit down. Remove gloves and any rings and undo her coat. Tell her to put her hands under her armpits to warm them with her own body heat.

Remove clothing from affected area carefully

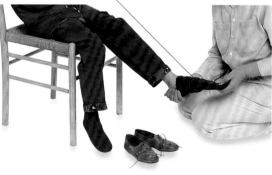

**2** Very gently remove her shoes and socks. Raise her feet to reduce swelling.

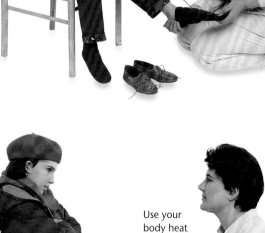

Use your body heat to thaw feet

**3** Place her feet in your own armpits to warm her toes.

**SEEK MEDICAL ADVICE**

# Heat exhaustion

This may develop in hot, humid weather or through physical exersion and is caused by dehydration. Children who are unwell, particularly with diarrhoea and vomiting, and those not used to the heat are most at risk. Suspect this if a child: complains of a headache, dizziness and nausea; is sweating; has pale, clammy skin; cramps; and a rapid, weakening pulse.

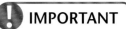
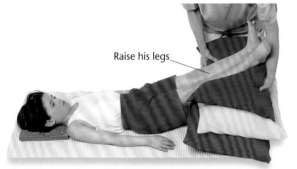

Lay child down in cool room

Put folded towel or cushion under his head

**1** Take your child into the shade or into a cool room. Help him to lie down.

Raise his legs

**2** Raise and support your child's legs on some pillows. This improves blood supply to the brain. Encourage him to rest quietly.

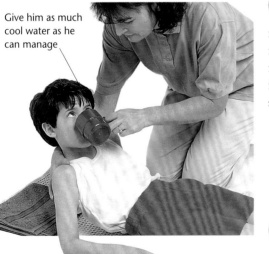

Give him as much cool water as he can manage

**3** Help your child to sit up and sip as much cool water as he can manage. Later give oral rehydration salts or an isotonic drink to replace salt lost from the body.

**SEEK MEDICAL ADVICE**

**》 see also**

● Heatstroke, *p.94*

● Unconscious baby, *pp.17–21*

● Unconscious child, *p.22–29*

## ! IMPORTANT

● **If** a baby or very young child develops heatstroke, undress him completely in a cool room.

● **If** your child loses consciousness, open his airway and check breathing. If breathing, place in the recovery position; if not breathing, begin rescue breaths and chest compressions.

# Heatstroke

This is a serious condition that develops if the body becomes overheated in hot surroundings. Treat for heatstroke if your child: develops a sudden headache; is confused; has hot, flushed, dry skin; has a full bounding pulse; is losing consciousness; has a temperature of over 40°C (104°F).

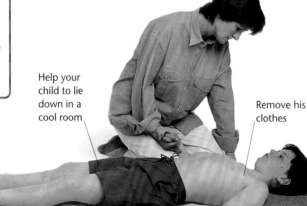

Help your child to lie down in a cool room

Remove his clothes

**1** Help your child to lie down in a cool place and remove all outer clothing. Put a folded towel or pillow under his head and reassure him.

☎ **CALL AN AMBULANCE**

Sponge his face and body with cold water

**2** Sponge down your child repeatedly with cold water. Ideally, wrap him in a cold, wet sheet.

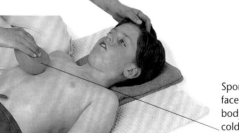

Cool him by fanning

**3** Fan your child by hand or with an electric fan to help bring his temperature down. Continue cooling until his temperature is down to 38°C (100.4°F).

## ≫ see also

● Unconscious baby, pp.17–21

● Unconscious child, p.22–29

# Sunburn

Sunburn is red, itchy, and tender. Babies and young children are very vulnerable: keep them in shade; apply sun block; put on a hat and cover with protective clothing in hot weather.

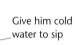

Give him cold water to sip

Apply cooling cream to reduce discomfort

**1** Move your child into the shade or into a cool room and give him a cold drink.

**2** Apply calamine cream or a special after-sun cream to soothe the skin. Make sure it is a cream that you *know* your child is not allergic to.

> **!** **IMPORTANT**
>
> ● **If** there is blistering, SEEK MEDICAL ADVICE.
>
> ● **If** your child is restless, flushed, dizzy, or has a temperature or headache, he may have heatstroke.

> **»** *see also*
>
> ● Heat exhaustion, *p.93*
> ● Heatstroke, *opposite*

# Heat rash

This a prickly, red rash that develops particularly around the sweat glands on the chest and back and under the arms.

**1** Help your child to sit down in a cool room and undress her. Sponge the affected area with cool water.

**2** Pat her almost dry with a soft towel, leaving the skin slightly damp. Apply calamine cream to the rash.

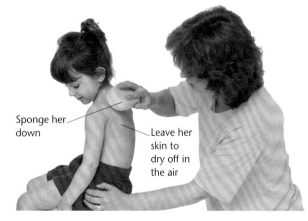

Sponge her down

Leave her skin to dry off in the air

> **!** **IMPORTANT**
>
> ● **If** your baby develops heat rash, remove some of her clothes to cool her, or bathe her in tepid water. Dry her gently, leaving her skin slightly damp.
>
> ● **If** the rash has not faded after 12 hours, or if she develops a raised temperature, SEEK MEDICAL ADVICE.

# Fever

A body temperature that is above 37°C (98.6°F) indicates fever. An infection is the usual cause. A moderate fever is not harmful, but a temperature above 40°C (104°F) can be dangerous, particularly in babies and very young children. Your child has a fever if she: has a raised temperature; looks very pale; complains she feels cold with goose pimples; is shivering, with chattering teeth. As the fever advances she will have hot, flushed skin, be sweating, and have a headache.

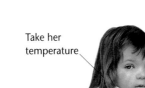

Take her temperature

Tuck the thermometer under her arm

**1** Take your child's temperature. If you are using a digital thermometer, lift your child's arm and tuck the pointed end into her armpit. Fold her arm over her chest and leave the thermometer in place for the recommended time.

**2** Make your child comfortable on a bed or sofa, but do not cover her. To help bring down her temperature, make sure she has plenty of water or diluted fruit juice to drink.

Leave a drink beside her

**3** You can give her the recommended dose of paracetamol syrup to help reduce her temperature.

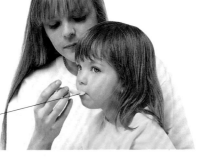

Give her the recommended dose of paracetamol syrup

>> *see also*

• Febrile seizures, *p.32*

• Heatstroke, *p.94*

• Meningitis, *opposite*

# Meningitis

This is a life-threatening infection affecting the tissues that surround the brain. In the early stages your child will have a flu-like illness with a high temperature. He may tell you he has cold hands and feet, joint and limb pain, and he may have mottled or very pale skin. As infection develops he is likely to have a headache, neck stiffness, and begin vomiting. His eyes may be sensitive to light and he will become increasingly drowsy. Later, a red or purple rash may develop that does not disappear if pressed.

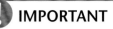

**IMPORTANT**

● **If** there is any delay contacting medical advice, TAKE YOUR CHILD TO HOSPITAL or CALL AN AMBULANCE.

● **Do not** let him get too hot.

● **In** some cases, the rash may not develop, or if it does, it will be one of the last symptoms to appear.

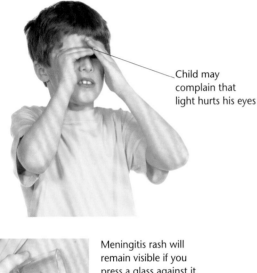

Child may complain that light hurts his eyes

**1** If your child has a high fever and a flu–like illness, monitor him carefully. If light hurts his eyes, let him rest in a darker room and monitor for other signs. Treat fever. Give him plenty of fluids to drink and the recommended dose of paracetamol syrup.

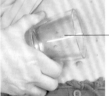

Meningitis rash will remain visible if you press a glass against it

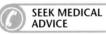
**SEEK MEDICAL ADVICE**

**2** Check your child's body for signs of a rash. If you see any spots, press a glass gently against them. If you can still see the spots through the glass.

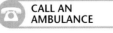
**CALL AN AMBULANCE**

Press side of a glass against the rash

**»** *see also*
● Febrile seizures, *p.32*
● Fever, *opposite*

# Vomiting and diarrhoea

A baby or child who is suffering repeated vomiting and/or diarrhoea can become dehydrated very quickly. It is important to replace lost fluids by giving your child sips of cooled, boiled water. Don't give a baby or child milk unless you are breastfeeding.

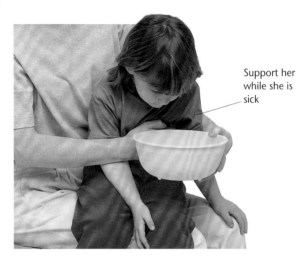

Support her while she is sick

**1** If your child is being sick, hold her over a bowl. Support her upper body with your free hand while she is being sick. Reassure her.

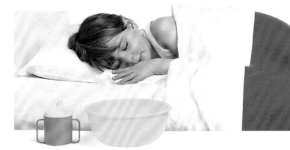

Give her water to drink

**2** Give her drinks of water to replace any fluid loss and to remove the unpleasant taste. Encourage her to sip each drink slowly.

**3** Let her rest quietly, in bed if she wants to. Make sure the bowl is still at hand in case she is sick again, and give a fresh drink of water.

# Stomachache

This is generally caused by a stomach upset as a result of an infection such as food poisoning.

**!  IMPORTANT**

● **If** the pain is severe, or does not subside after 30 minutes, SEEK MEDICAL ADVICE.

● **If** your child has been "winded", sit her down and loosen clothing around her waist. The pain should ease quickly. If in you are in any doubt, SEEK MEDICAL ADVICE.

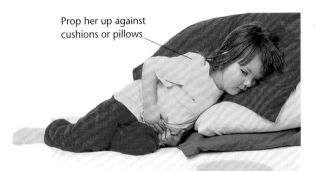

Prop her up against cushions or pillows

**1** Make your child comfortable on a sofa or bed. Help her to lie back against cushions or pillows. She may want to be sick so leave a container near her.

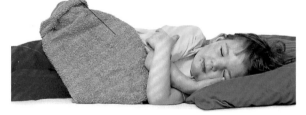

Give her a covered hot-water bottle to hold

**2** Warmth may help to relieve the pain. Fill a hot-water bottle – it must be covered – and give it to your child to hold against her stomach. Avoid giving her anything to eat until pain subsides.

## Appendicitis

Suspect appendicitis if your child complains of waves of pain in the middle of his abdomen or of acute pain settling in the right lower abdomen. He may also have a raised temperature, no appetite, nausea, vomiting, and diarrhoea.

Suspected appendicitis must be treated promptly. Help your child to lie down. Do not give him anything to eat or drink.

Pain starts here

Pain settles here

**SEEK MEDICAL ADVICE**

**! IMPORTANT**

● **If** pain does not begin to subside, or if there is a discharge from the ear, fever, or hearing loss, SEEK MEDICAL ADVICE.

# Earache

This is most commonly caused by an ear infection following a cold or flu. Earache can be the result of a child putting something in her ear.

## Pressure-change earache

This may happen on plane journeys, particularly when taking off or landing, or when travelling through tunnels. To make the ears "pop" so that the pressure is relieved, an older child should close her mouth, hold her nose and blow down it. Sucking a sweet may also help.

Give her recommended dose of paracetamol syrup

**1** Make your child comfortable. Help her to sit up supported by pillows or cushions if lying down makes the earache worse. You can give the recommended dose of paracetamol syrup.

**2** Applying heat may help to soothe the pain. Prepare a covered hot-water bottle and tell your child to lie down with her painful ear against it.

Provide a covered hot-water bottle to place against her ear

Prop her up with pillows

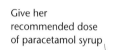

# Toothache

A toddler who complains of toothache may have a new tooth coming through. An older child may have tooth decay or an infection.

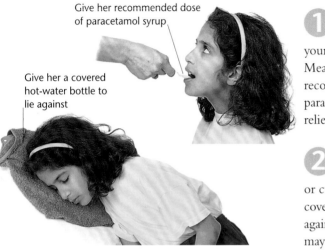

Give her recommended dose of paracetamol syrup

Give her a covered hot-water bottle to lie against

**1** Arrange an early appointment with your child's dentist. Meanwhile, give her the recommended dose of paracetamol syrup to relieve the pain.

**2** Lying flat, or propped on pillows or cushions, with a covered hot-water bottle against the affected cheek may help relieve the pain.

# Cramp

Cramp is a painful muscle spasm that often affects the foot and calf muscles. You can relieve the pain by massaging and stretching the affected muscles.

**1** Help your child to sit down then raise her leg and straighten her knee. Ease her toes upwards to flex the foot.

**2** Gently but firmly knead the affected muscles with your fingertips until the spasm has passed completely.

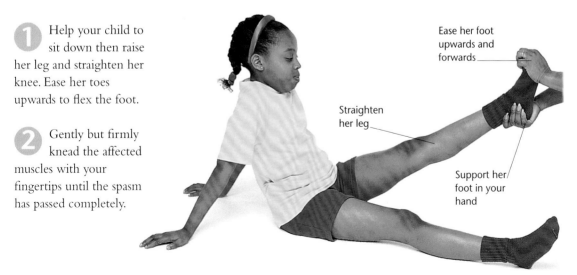

Ease her foot upwards and forwards

Straighten her leg

Support her foot in your hand

## A well-stocked first aid kit

- Disposable gloves
- Small roller bandage
- Large roller bandage
- Small conforming bandage
- Large conforming bandage
- Blunt-ended scissors
- Plastic tweezers
- Pack of gauze swabs
- Triangular bandages
- Hypoallergenic tape
- Sterile non-adhesive pads
- Waterproof plasters
- Sterile dressings

# First aid kit

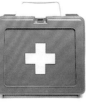

Keep first aid kits in your car and in your home. You can buy kits ready made up. You may want to add extra dressings and bandages or specialist plasters – blister plasters, for example. Make sure the first aid box is readily accessible and easy to identify, and check the contents regularly. Do not keep medicines in the same box; they should be locked in a medicine cabinet. A well-stocked kit might contain the articles shown here. *See p.108* for alternative household items.

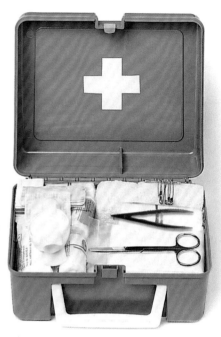

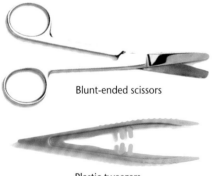

Blunt-ended scissors

Plastic tweezers

## Dressings

Plasters (adhesive dressings) are used for minor wounds. Keep several different sizes and shapes, including a selection of larger sterile dressings for more serious wounds.

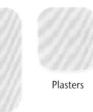

Plasters

Gauze swabs

Sterile non-adhesive pad

Sterile dressing with bandage attached

# Bandages

Keep a variety of bandages to secure dressings and support injured joints. Conforming bandages shape themselves to the contours of the body and so are easy to use. Triangular bandages can be used as slings and for broad- and narrow-fold bandages.

Tape for securing dressings

Small conforming bandage

Large conforming bandage

Clip secures bandage

Crepe roller bandage

Large roller bandage

Safety pins

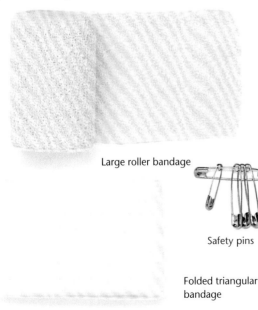

Folded triangular bandage

# Additional useful equipment

- If you have a note pad and pen or pencil you can write down important information about a child's condition to give to the emergency services.
- Keep a torch beside your home first aid kit (for use in the event of a power failure), and in your car; check and replace the batteries regularly.
- Plastic face shields or face masks can protect you and a child when you are giving rescue breaths.
- Keep a plastic or foil emergency survival blanket or bag in your car.
- Always carry a warning triangle in your car and place it in the road behind the car in the event of a breakdown or crash.

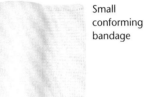

## REHYDRATION SALTS

Sachets of rehydration salts are added to water. Use them to treat dehydration resulting from heat exhaustion or vomiting.

## INSTANT ICE PACKS

Keep a pack of these in the home or car – they are especially useful when you do not have access to a freezer.

## DIGITAL THERMOMETER

Choose one with an easy-to-read screen. Check the battery regularly.

# Dressings

Covering a wound helps the blood-clotting process and prevents infection. Dressings should not be fluffy and must be large enough to cover the wound and area around it. Wash your hands before applying dressings and wear disposable gloves if possible. If blood soaks through a dressing, place another on top. Make sure bandages are not too tight (*see opposite*).

## Plaster

Remove wrapping and, holding the pad over the wound, peel back the protective strips. Press the ends and edges down.

## Sterile pad

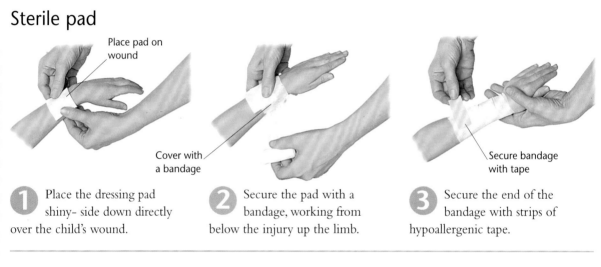

Place pad on wound

Cover with a bandage

Secure bandage with tape

**1** Place the dressing pad shiny- side down directly over the child's wound.

**2** Secure the pad with a bandage, working from below the injury up the limb.

**3** Secure the end of the bandage with strips of hypoallergenic tape.

## Sterile dressing with bandage

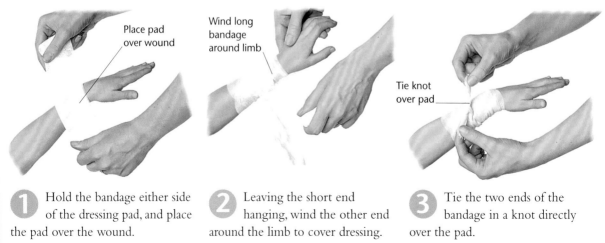

Place pad over wound

Wind long bandage around limb

Tie knot over pad

**1** Hold the bandage either side of the dressing pad, and place the pad over the wound.

**2** Leaving the short end hanging, wind the other end around the limb to cover dressing.

**3** Tie the two ends of the bandage in a knot directly over the pad.

# Bandaging

Use bandages to secure dressings, to help control bleeding, and to support injuries. Roller bandages can be used for any part of the body; conforming bandages are especially useful for bandaging joints or head wounds as they mould themselves to the shape of the body.

## Check circulation

Do not apply a bandage too tightly – it will impair the circulation. To check, press on your child's nail or a patch of skin, then release pressure. The colour should return rapidly. If it does not, loosen the bandages.

## Roller bandage

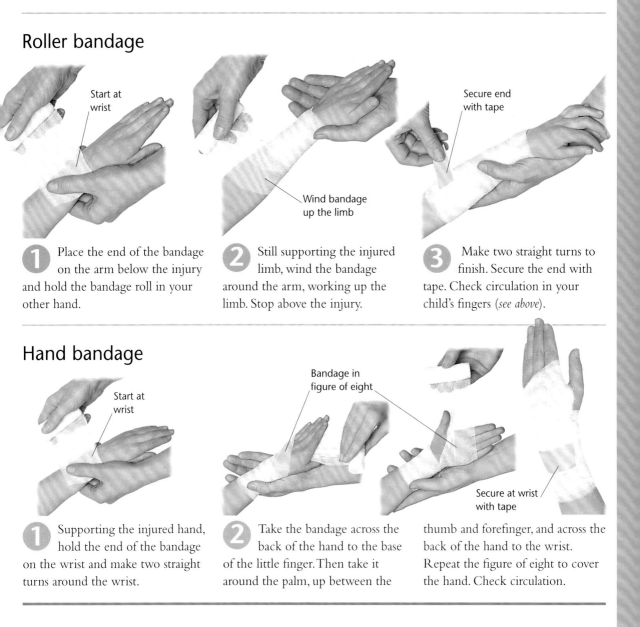

Start at wrist

Wind bandage up the limb

Secure end with tape

**1** Place the end of the bandage on the arm below the injury and hold the bandage roll in your other hand.

**2** Still supporting the injured limb, wind the bandage around the arm, working up the limb. Stop above the injury.

**3** Make two straight turns to finish. Secure the end with tape. Check circulation in your child's fingers (*see above*).

## Hand bandage

Start at wrist

Bandage in figure of eight

Secure at wrist with tape

**1** Supporting the injured hand, hold the end of the bandage on the wrist and make two straight turns around the wrist.

**2** Take the bandage across the back of the hand to the base of the little finger. Then take it around the palm, up between the

thumb and forefinger, and across the back of the hand to the wrist. Repeat the figure of eight to cover the hand. Check circulation.

# Triangular bandages

These are sold singly in sterile packs or can be made from a square of strong fabric folded diagonally in half. Triangular bandages are used for broad-fold and narrow-fold bandages (*see p.73*) or slings. Arm slings support injured arms or wrists, or take weight off an injured shoulder. Elevation slings are used to suppport hand injuries to minimise bleeding, pain, or swelling.

## Arm sling

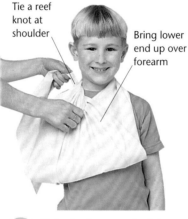

Drape long edge of triangle on uninjured side

Tie a reef knot at shoulder

Bring lower end up over forearm

Make sure the knot is comfortable

Tuck in surplus fabric at elbow

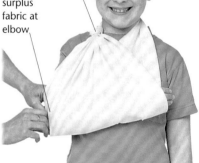

**1** Place the bandage between your child's arm and chest, easing one end up around the back of his neck on the injured side.

**2** Take the lower end of the bandage up over your child's forearm to the end at the shoulder and tie a knot just below the shoulder.

**3** Fold in the surplus fabric at the corner near the elbow and pin it to the bandage.

## Improvised slings

If your child injures her shoulder, arm, or hand, you can make an improvised sling to support the injury until she receives medical treatment.

● Undo a coat or shirt button and tuck the hand of the injured arm inside the fastening.

● Pin your child's sleeve up on the opposite side of his chest.

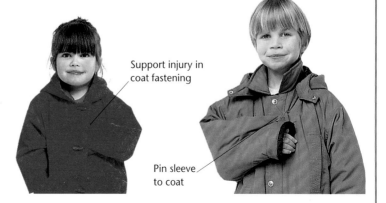

Support injury in coat fastening

Pin sleeve to coat

# Elevation sling

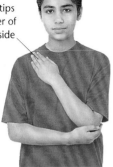

Rest fingertips on shoulder of uninjured side

**1** Bring the arm on the injured side across your child's chest. Ask her to support her elbow.

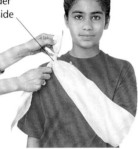

Hold top corner at shoulder

Drape long edge across body

**2** Lay bandage over child's arm, with longest edge on the uninjured side. Hold the top corner.

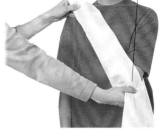

Scoop bandage up around elbow

**3** Support the child's arm and fold long edge of bandage in under injured arm.

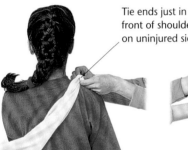

Tie ends just in front of shoulder on uninjured side

**4** Bring the lower end up around her back, holding the elbow securely in the fabric. Tie a knot just below the shoulder and tuck the ends in.

Gather slack fabric at elbow and tuck in behind

**OR**

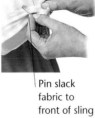

Pin slack fabric to front of sling

**5** Secure the sling by twisting the excess fabric and tucking it in at the elbow or fold and pin in place.

Finished sling raises, immobilises, and supports the injury

# Useful household items

You should keep a well-stocked first aid kit (*see p.102*) at home and in the car. However, there are many everyday items around the home that are invaluable for first aid emergencies.

- Plastic credit cards can be used to scrape off an insect sting (*see p.86*).
- A tea towel can be used as a pad to control bleeding or as an improvised dressing or to secure a dressing.
- Use vinegar to treat a jellyfish sting (*see p.88*) – it neutralises the effect of the sting and prevents it from spreading.
- Beer or milk can be used to cool a burn if there is no cold water available (*see p.58*).
- Milk stops a knocked-out adult tooth drying out while you get the child to a dentist (*see p.53*).
- Use a telephone directory, thick book, or wooden box as insulation when dealing with electrical injury (*see p.12*).

## Making a cold compress

- Packs of frozen vegetables such as peas or fruit such as raspberries or currants wrapped in a tea towel make ideal ice packs. The bags mould to the shape of the body and stay cool for a long time.

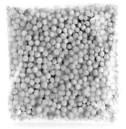

- Fill a sandwich or freezer bag two-thirds full of ice cubes, then seal the bag. Wrap it in a tea towel before putting on your child.

Frozen peas in a plastic bag

- Soak a flannel in water, wring out the excess water, then place it over the injury.

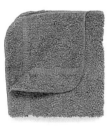

### FLANNEL
Use a flannel soaked in water to make a cold compress as well as clean up a child after an incident.

### PLASTIC BAGS
A clean plastic bag can be put over a burned foot or hand and lightly secured with bandages or tape. Always cool the burn first.

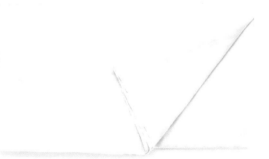

### SHEETS AND PILLOW CASES
A clean cotton sheet or pillowcase makes an excellent loose protective covering for burns.

### CLING FILM
Plastic kitchen film can be used to cover burns and seal chest wounds.

# Safety at home

Most accidents occur at home and over half involve children under the age of five. Many accidents are preventable if you:

- Plan the layout and position of objects and furniture at home with child safety in mind.
- Make sure that all windows are closed or inaccessible (don't leave chairs beside them).
- Never confuse containers by putting a dangerous substance, such as bleach, in a bottle that used to contain a harmless drink.
- Install smoke alarms, carbon monoxide alarms, fire guards, and safety gates in your home.
- Never pretend that medicines and pills are special sweets to encourage a child to take medication. Keep medicines locked away.
- Check for hazards when visiting friends and ask if you can move sharp or breakable objects.
- Teach your child basic safety rules.

## Fire

If fire breaks out at home, it could be a matter of minutes before smoke overcomes you.

- Fit smoke alarms throughout your home. If your home is on one level, fit a detector between the sitting room and the bedrooms. If your house is on two or more levels, fit one detector at the foot of the stairs and another on every floor outside the bedrooms. If you live in an apartment block there should be detectors in all communal areas as well.
- Check smoke alarms regularly; replace batteries if they have them.
- Have an escape plan (*see p. 11*). Make sure the whole family knows what to do if there is a fire, especially at night. Practise the fire drill with your children:

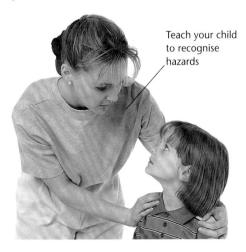

Teach your child to recognise hazards

shout "fire"; tell everyone to drop to the floor if there is smoke and crawl to the nearest exit from the rooms; shut each door behind you; arrange a point outside where everyone should wait together.

- Don't go back for pets or treasured possessions.

## Electricity

Protect your child from electric shock (*see p. 12*) or fire caused by electric faults.

- Cover sockets: put heavy furniture in front of them.
- Use bar-type fused adaptors on extension leads instead of block-type socket adaptors.
- Wire plugs correctly – follow instructions and check that you have the right fuse.
- Replace worn or damaged flexes.
- Tidy up trailing wires to prevent tripping hazards.
- Unplug electrical appliances at night, particularly the televisions and computers.
- Fit an RCD (residual current device) to power tools.

## Gas

Find out where your gas tap is in case there is a leak. If you smell gas call 0800 111 999:

- Don't turn lights or electric switches on or off – there may be a spark, which can cause an explosion.
- Don't light matches or cigarettes.
- Turn off the gas and open the windows.
- Fit carbon monoxide alarms and have all boilers and gas appliances serviced regularly.

# Hall and stairs

The staircase is not a safe place for your child to play (*see below*).

- Make sure that toys are not left on the stairs for you to trip over.
- Put a light in your hall or on the landing so that your child can see if he gets up at night.

If you don't want the area too light, use a low-watt bulb. Never cover a lamp with a cloth as the cloth can easily catch fire.

- Don't let your child play on the landings or stairs of a communal area in flats as the banisters may have large gaps between them.

## Front and back doors

- Never leave your front door open.
- Don't let your child answer the door to callers.
- Put the door catch out of reach of small children. If your toddler can reach the catch, fix an additional bolt higher up the door and keep the door bolted.
- If the door has a deadlick that needs a key to open, the key needs to be accessible to adults and older children so that they can escape in the event of a fire.
- Stick plastic safety film over glass doors if the glass is within 80cm (2ft 8in) of the floor; this prevents the glass splintering if it is broken. Better still, fit toughened or laminated glass.
- Put stickers over the glass to make it more noticeable, especially for young children.

## Floors

Tiled, polished, or hessian-covered floors can be very slippery for toddlers and running children.

- Put non-slip webbing under rugs.
- Keep hall floors free of toys and clutter.
- Check fitted carpets regularly for holes or loose carpet that might trip you or your toddler.

## Stairs

A child is not coordinated enough to be able to walk downstairs safely until he is at least three years old.

- Fit safety gates at the foot of the stairs and across the upper landing or across your child's bedroom doorway (safety gates at the top of the stairs can be a trip hazard). Safety gates should comply with British Standard EN 1930:2011 so the bars are no more than

6.5cm (2½ in) apart. Always open the gate; never climb over it as your child will copy you.

- Check your banisters regularly: the handrail and posts should be secured. Posts should not be too far apart – anything wider than 6.5cm (2½ in) apart should be boarded up. Don't let your child climb banisters. If the guarding on stairs or landing is made of horizontal rails (so-called ranch-type banisters), it should be boarded up because it is very easy for a child to climb them.
- Replace loose or worn carpet or steps. They are trip hazards.

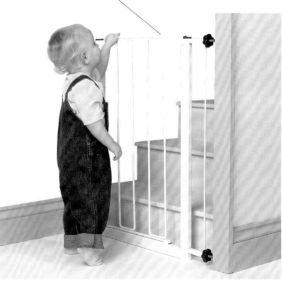

Keep the safety gate closed

# Sitting room

While your children are very young, try to arrange the room so that both children and your valuables are kept out of harm's way.

- If you have a balcony, block up gaps in the railings with hardboard and ensure that the balcony is too high for your child to climb.
- Fit safety glass in patio doors if the glass is within 80cm (2ft 8in) of the floor.

## Carpets and curtains

- Check that there are no areas of carpet or rug that have holes or turned-up edges; either you or your child could trip up.
- Wind up and tuck away all curtain ties and pull cords for blinds. Children can be strangled if they get caught in dangling cords.

## Fireplaces and heaters

- Don't leave matches or cigarette lighters where your child can reach them.
- Cover all fires with a fireguard. Fix the guard to the wall to prevent your child pulling it over.
- Use a spark-guard as well as a fireguard for open solid fuel fires as an additional precaution.
- Never use the fireguard as a shelf or clothes airer.

## Electrical equipment

- Fix wiring to the skirting board.
- Run long flexes behind furniture so that your child can't trip or pull on them.
- Check that old flexes are not worn.
- Ensure that the TV stand is secure and cannot be pulled over. Flat screen TVs should be attached to the wall.

## Surfaces and furniture

- Place house plants out of reach of young children. Some house plants are poisonous, and others can scratch or produce allergic reactions if touched.
- Do not place breakable or heavy objects on low tables. Set them well back from the edges of surfaces such as window sills or mantelpieces.
- Glass-topped tables should comply with BS EN 12521:2009. Put protectors on sharp table corners.
- Don't leave hot drinks, alcohol, glasses, cigarettes, matches, or lighters on low surfaces, such as coffee tables, where your child can reach them.
- Keep alcohol in a locked cupboard.
- Never leave a cigarette burning in an ashtray on the arm of a sofa or armchair.
- Replace old foam furniture; it can be lethal in a fire as it releases toxic fumes as soon as it is alight.

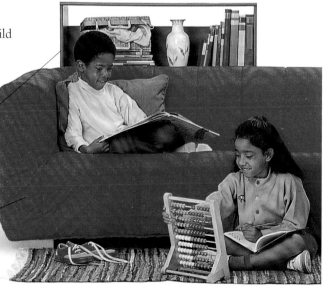

Ensure bookcases are secured to the wall

Sofas and armchairs must have fire-resistant fillings and coverings

# Kitchen

This is the busiest part of your house, where you spend a lot of time with your children.

- Never hold baby or child in your arms when you are cooking or carrying a hot drink.

## Doors

- Cover any glass panels within 80cm (2ft 8in) of the floor with safety film, to stop glass shattering or splintering if broken. Or fit safety glass.
- Put some colourful stickers on the glass door panels to alert your child.

## Floors

- Don't let your child play on the area of floor between you and the work surface or where you could trip over him.
- Avoid bumps and falls by wiping up spills immediately.
- Remove pet food bowls after use and keep that part of the floor scrupulously clean.
- Keep a box for tidying away toys and clutter.

## Wastebins

- Discourage toddlers from rummaging in the wastebin.
- Put sharp-edged cans and lids or broken glass straight into the dustbin outside.
- Keep the wastebin in a cupboard with a child-resistant safety catch.

> ### ! IMPORTANT
>
> - Keep a fire blanket in the kitchen for smothering flare-ups. If you want to buy a fire extinguisher, consult your local fire brigade to find out which is the most appropriate type. Check them regularly. For more on fires, *see p.11 and p.109.*

## Babies in the kitchen

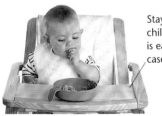

Stay with your child when he is eating in case he chokes

### BOTTLES AND FOOD

- Sterilise all your baby's feeding equipment, or put it in a dishwasher.
- Don't leave a prepared feed standing at room temperature, and don't keep the remains of the last feed. Warmed and reheated feeds are breeding grounds for bacteria.
- If you heat bottles, make sure you shake throughly and check the temperature before you feed your baby.

### HIGHCHAIRS

- Always use the safety harness.
- Never leave the chair where your baby can reach out and pull objects down from a surface.
- Never leave your child unattended in a highchair.

### PLAY

- Put your baby in a playpen away from the cooking area, or put a gate across the doorway so he can see you but is out of harm's way.
- Keep him out of range of any spills from the cooker.

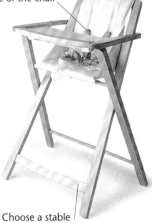

Attach a safety harness to the clips on either side of the chair

Choose a stable highchair with widely spaced legs

# Tables and work surfaces

- Always be aware of your child's reach and keep all heavy, breakable, or sharp objects well back from the edges of work surfaces.
- Keep stools or chairs away from tables and kitchen work surfaces to prevent a young child from climbing up on them.
- Tuck flexes of kettles, toasters, blenders, and irons out of reach. Choose a curly flex for your kettle if possible. It is not only boiling, steaming kettles that pose a hazard: the water in a kettle is still hot enough to scald 15 minutes after boiling.
- Leave electrical appliances unplugged when they are not in use.
- Avoid using a tablecloth. It is tempting for a crawling baby or toddler to use it to pull himself up, bringing anything on the table down upon his head. Use table mats instead, or secure the cloth with clips.
- Do not put your baby on a table or work surface when he is in a car seat or bouncing cradle: he could easily fall off.

# Cupboards and drawers

- Put safety catches on cupboards and drawers, particularly those containing: matches, lighters, knives, scissors, and cutlery; heavy pots, pans, or china; dried food, such as lentils or pasta, which may be a choking hazard; bottles containing alcohol; medicines; cleaning materials, such as washing powder, or dishwasher detergent, even if fitted with "child-resistant" lids.

# Fridges

Food poisoning can be caused by poor food storage. Take precautions to minimise risks:
- Keep cooked meat and poultry on a separate shelf from uncooked meat. Cover uncooked meat with kitchen film.
- Don't store food in open tins; tip leftovers into a clean container, cover, and put in the fridge.
- Check food regularly to see that nothing is kept beyond the "use-by" date.

# Cookers

Your child is obviously at risk of burns and scalds from hot fat or boiling water when you are preparing food.
- You can buy safety guards, but remember that a child can still poke fingers through some types and be burnt by hot hobs or gas rings.
- Always keep your child away from oven doors; they can get very hot while the oven is in use and will stay hot for some time afterwards. A crawling baby or toddler is particularly at risk. Try to teach your child what "hot" means so that he understands a warning.
- Keep matches and lighters well out of reach in a cupboard fitted with a safety catch.

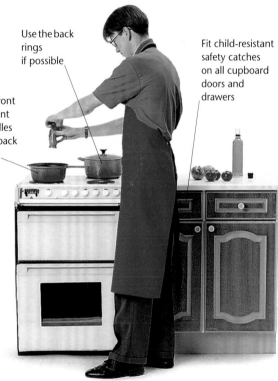

Use the back rings if possible

Fit child-resistant safety catches on all cupboard doors and drawers

If using front rings, point pan handles towards back of cooker

# Washing and drying machines

- Keep small hands away from the glass door; it may get hot while the machine is on.
- Ensure the door is closed when the machines are not in use. Your toddler may try to climb inside or even fill it with toys.

# Bedrooms

The cupboards and drawers in bedrooms are always exciting places for toddlers and young children. Make sure any potentially hazardous items are out of reach, as you may not always know when your child will decide to go exploring on his own.

## Baby's cots

- Make sure the cot is deep enough to prevent your baby from climbing out – at least 50cm (1ft 8in) from the top of the mattress to the top of the cot.

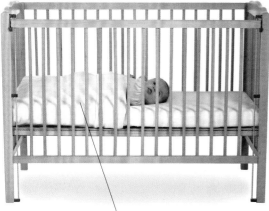

Put your baby down to sleep with his feet at the base of the cot

- Bar spaces must be between 2.5 and 6cm (1–2½in) wide to prevent your baby's head from being trapped.
- The mattress must fit the cot with a gap of less than 3cm (1½in) around the side or the baby's head could become trapped between the cot side and the mattress.
- Don't use a cot that has been handed down through generations; it is unlikely to meet safety standards.
- Don't use a pillow for a baby under one year: it could suffocate him. If you need to raise his head, put a pillow underneath the mattress.
- Use a sheet and cellular blankets rather than a duvet until your baby is one year old. Your baby could overheat or suffocate under a duvet.
- Always put your baby to sleep on his back with his feet at the foot of the cot to lessen the risk of cot death.
- Remove toys from the cot as soon as your baby can sit up because he could use them to climb out.
- Once your child starts trying to climb out of the cot, transfer him to a bed.

## Changing areas

- Keep all changing equipment in one area so that you never have to leave your baby alone on the changing mat. He will be safest on the floor, but if you have a changing table, remember that he might roll off if left even for a moment.
- Store nappy sacs well out of the reach of babies as these present a suffocation risk.
- Do not have shelves above the changing area in case something falls off onto your child.
- Keep dangling mobiles out of his reach.
- If you use talcum powder, sprinkle it on your hands and rub them together before applying it to avoid creating a cloud of dust around your baby.

Change your baby on the floor on a changing mat so that he cannot fall

# Children's bedrooms

This is a room where where children are likely to be unsupervised so they have to be as safe as possible.

- Stow blind and curtain cords well out of children's reach. Many blinds have cords built into them as part of their structure – Venetian blinds, for example – and these also pose a hazard. If buying blinds for a child's room, buy ones that do not have cords to operate them or within their structure.
- Don't use a bed guard when your toddler first moves to a bed; if you think he may fall out, put cushions on the floor beside the bed.
- A top bunk bed is not recommended for children under the age of six.
- Top bunk beds must have safety rails on both sides and any gaps in the railings or between the top of the mattress and the bottom of the safety rail should be no more than 6–7.5cm (2½–3in).
- Never let young children play on the top bunk.
- Remove toys from the floor by the bed at night.
- Ensure no wires the child can pull are near bed.

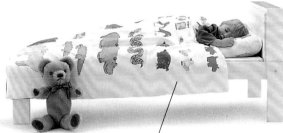

Avoid feather pillows and duvets as they can provoke allergies

## WINDOWS

Make sure your child can't climb out of the window. He is in danger even if his room is on the ground floor.

- Fix a safety catch, but make sure the window can be opened easily in the event of a fire.
- Try not to place a piece of furniture below a window because it may encourage your child to climb up.

## TOYS *(see also p.117)*

- Keep toys that are unsuitable for very young children separate from others. This way you can easily put them out of reach if your child is sharing a room with a younger child, or if you have young visitors.

Put non-slip webbing under rugs

# Your bedroom

The Foudation for the Study of Infant Deaths (FSID) advises that babies under 6 months should sleep in a cot, and not in a parent's bed.

- Medicines and pills should never be left beside your bed, or on a dressing table. Put them out of sight and out of reach, preferably in a locked cupboard.
- Scissors and sewing equipment should be kept in a drawer or cupboard with a safety catch.
- Perfume, hairspray, and makeup can be harmful if sprayed or rubbed in the eyes, or swallowed, so keep them out of reach or in a drawer with a safety catch. Make-up spills can also stain a carpet.
- Never leave a china cup or a glass on the floor by your bed, especially at night. If your child is in your bed he could roll out onto the cup or the glass.

# Bathroom

Your child may be at risk from falls, drowning, scalding, or poisoning in the bathroom. Keep the door shut at all times to discourage him from going in. If you install a bolt to the door, fix it towards the top of the door to prevent a young child locking himself in.

## Baths

- Check the temperature of the water before your child gets into the bath. Put your elbow in the water; if it is too hot for your elbow it is too hot for your child. A child can be badly scalded by hot bathwater.
- Fit thermostatic mixing valves to the hot taps to limit the temperature of water from the tap.
- Place non-slip mats in the bath and on the floor beside the bath.
- Keep babies and toddlers away from the bath taps.
- Never leave a young child or baby alone in the bath (or in the care of another child). A baby can drown in just 2.5cm (1in) of water. If you need to answer the door or telephone, take your baby with you.

## Showers

- Keep a constant check on the temperature of the water.
- Use non-slip mats in the shower and on the bathroom floor.
- Fix safety film on a glass shower door so that glass is held in place in case of an accident.

## Cupboards and cabinets

- Store bathroom chemicals and other potential poisons, such as toilet cleaners and bleach, out of reach in a cupboard with a safety catch.
- Keep other hazards, such as make-up, aftershave, razors, nail scissors, and any medicines or glass containers, out of reach in a locked medicine cabinet.

## Toilets

- Use a special child toilet seat adaptor and step for toddlers so that they can keep their balance more easily and so feel more secure.
- Keep the toilet seat closed.
- Don't use block toilet cleaners that a young child could pull out and chew.
- Never use toilet cleaners as well as bleach as this will produce toxic fumes.
- If your toddler uses a potty, keep it clean, but never leave bleach or cleaning agents inside it.

Bath him away from the taps

Use a non-slip mat in the bath

# Toys and playthings

If you have children of different ages in your home, keep their toys in separate boxes. In particular, keep toys with small parts away from younger children.

## Choosing toys

- Buy toys that are appropriate for the age of your child, and buy from a reputable source.
- Don't give your child anything to play with that has sharp edges, or is made of thin, rigid plastic.
- Give him non-toxic paints or crayons.
- Don't buy your child old second-hand toys: they may be broken or covered in paint containing lead.
- Avoid novelty toys that are not designed to be played with by young children: look out for warnings on the packaging.

Give your child non-toxic paints to play with

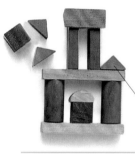

Check sets of building blocks for small pieces that could be a choking hazard for a younger child

## Caring for toys

- Check toys regularly and always throw away any broken ones.
- Don't mix old and new batteries. Change them all at the same time, otherwise the strong batteries will make the weak ones very hot.
- Keep toys in a toy box. Toys can bring about accidents or injuries if left on the floor.

## Babies and toddlers

- Remove ribbons from a baby's soft toys.
- Check that the eyes, noses, ears, or bells on soft toys and dolls are well secured.
- Attach cot toys with a very short string and remove them as soon as your baby can sit up.
- Remove activity centres or bulky toys from a cot as soon as your child can stand because they provide a foothold for climbing out of the cot.
- Don't let babies chew on furry toys: the fur is a choking hazard.
- Never let a young child play with a toy that is not recommended for his age-group: it may contain small pieces on which he could choke.
- Don't leave baby or toddler to play in a room on his own.
- Baby walkers serve no useful purpose. If you

do use one, make sure it complies with BS EN 1273: 2005. Older walkers can tip over, and can be dangerous for your baby.

Make sure that toys that increase mobility are stable

# Garden

Your garden can be a safe and interesting place for your children to play. Children will find their own corners to play in but you must clear away rubbish and remove obvious hazards:

- Lock gates that lead out of the garden and make sure fences are secure.

- Check garden furniture or play equipment regularly to make sure that it is stable and safe. Site it over grass not paving stones.
- Keep pets off areas where children play.
- Make sure paving is even and remove moss: children may easily trip or slip.

## Plants

Many plants are poisonous if eaten and digested in large quantities. Small pieces, or one or two berries, are not fatal but may cause some discomfort and stomach upset.

- Tell your child about the dangers of eating berries, and keep babies and toddlers away from them.
- Remove plants that you know to be poisonous, such as deadly nightshade, laburnum, and toadstools.
- Cut back any prickly plants, such as roses, brambles, and holly. They can give nasty scratches, especially to your or your child's eyes.

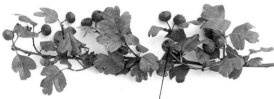

Warn your child not to eat berries or leaves

## Sheds

Sheds are inevitably used for storing chemical and tools. and so are a potential hazard.

- Tell your child that the shed is out of bounds, keep it locked at all times, and hide the key.
- Put any chemicals, such as weedkiller or slug pellets, out of reach in containers with child-resistant tops.

## Water in the garden

Babies and toddlers are especially at risk if they slip and fall, even in shallow water. Maintain fencing to prevent children entering a neighbour's garden where a pond may be a hazard.

- Never leave children unattended when they are playing in, or near, water.
- Keep ponds covered and fenced off, and cover water butts and empty dustbins that collect rainwater.
- Always empty out a paddling pool when your children have finished playing in it and turn it upside-down in case it rains.

## Gardening

- Don't put down chemicals when children will be playing in the garden.
- Don't mow the lawn while children are close by because stone chips may become dislodged and fly up into their eyes.
- Put away all garden tools when you have finished using them.

Check that he is playing in a clean, safe area with safe toys

# Garage and car safety

Always leave your garage locked; likewise keep the car locked, even if it is on a driveway off the road or in a garage. Keep the car keys where the children cannot reach them. Don't give the keys to your baby to play with as they are not clean and he could drop them.

## Garages and drives

- Keep the garage locked and discourage your child from going in there.
- Keep equipment, chemicals, or tools out of your child's reach and locked away if possible.
- Make sure you know where your child is when you are driving into, or out of, the garage or a drive.
- If you keep a deep freeze in the garage, it should be locked at all times.

## Cars

- Never leave a young child unattended in a car, even if you can see the car.
- Don't let your child play with the car windows, whether manual or electric. Windows can trap a child's head or fingers.
- Remove the cigarette lighter from the car altogether.
- Watch out for your child's fingers when you shut the car doors.
- Use child locks on rear doors until your child is at least six years old.
- Teach your child to get out of the car on the pavement side.
- If your child is helping you wash the car, make sure you have removed the car keys from the ignition first.

## Car seats

Always put your child into a special safety seat when you strap him into the car. The law requires that all children up to 135cm (about 4ft 5in) travelling in cars use a child restraint. You should never carry a child on your lap – it is dangerous and illegal.

There are various types of car seat – the correct one will depend on the age or your baby or child and your car.

Ideally when you buy a seat, go to a retailer who will allow you to try it in your car before you buy it, and who will show you how to use it properly. Fit the seat exactly as the instructions describe.

Choose the correct seat for the weight and development of your child:

- Babies up to 13kg (29lb) – about 12–15 months – should travel in a rear-facing car seat. The baby is harnessed into the seat and the seat is held in place by the car seat belts. The safest place for your baby to travel is on the rear seat of your car. Do not place your baby in a rear-facing car seat on the front passenger seat if there is an airbag fitted – the impact of an airbag inflating could cause serious injury.
- Never hold a baby on your lap or inside your own seatbelt: he would be thrown out of the car or crushed by your body weight in a crash.
- Older babies and toddlers, up to 18kg (40lb), need a car seat in the back of the car. Some seats have an integral harness for the child, which fits over his shoulders, across his hips, and between his legs. The seats are held in place by the adult seat belt, or straps that you fix into the car. Other types of seat use the adult belt to restrain both the child and the seat. Most new cars have special ISOFIX seat fixings for child car seats.
- As a child gets bigger, he or she should travel in a booster seat. Without it, adult seat belts are neither comfortable nor safe: the shoulder part cuts across the child's neck, and the lap strap lies across his stomach, which could cause internal injury in a crash. A lap strap on its own is not sufficient as it does not restrain the child's upper body.

Finally, use the seat on every journey, no matter how short.

# Out and about

After the home, most childhood accidents occur in the street or in play areas. Teach your child the rules of the road from an early age, reminding him to stay alert for traffic and to cross in a safe place. It takes a long time for children to develop a true road sense.

## What a child understands
- Three-year-olds can learn that the pavement is safe and the road is dangerous.
- Five-year-olds can learn how to cross the road, but they are still not able to put this knowledge into practice on their own.
- Eight-year-olds can cross quiet streets on their own, but they are not yet able to judge the speed and distance of traffic.
- Twelve-year-olds can judge the speed of an oncoming car, but are still easily distracted by friends.

## Street and road safety
Whenever you are out with your child, show him how to be aware of his own safety.
- When out shopping or walking near a road, use reins or a wrist strap for a toddler, to stop him running off without you.
- Encourage a young child to hold your hand when you are near the road or waiting to cross a road.

## Learning how to cross the road
Teach your child the rules of the road:
- Find a safe place to cross, then stop.
- Stand on the pavement, near the kerb.
- Look all around for traffic, and listen.
- If traffic is coming, let it pass.
- When there is no traffic near, walk straight across the road.
- Look and listen for traffic while you cross.

- Teach your child by example and always find a safe place to cross a road. This may be a zebra crossing, a pelican crossing with lights, an underpass, or a footbridge. If there is no designated crossing point, aim for a large gap between parked cars, where you and your child can see a long way in both directions.
- At a zebra crossing teach your child to stop and wait until all the traffic has stopped and to stop at the island halfway across, if there is one.
- When using a pelican crossing at traffic lights, encourage your child to press the button and always wait until the traffic has stopped before crossing.

## Bikes
- Children under 10 years old should not cycle on roads in traffic without an adult and all children should have cycle training before going on the road.
- Make sure your child can be seen when he's riding his bike – with bright fluorescent colours by day and reflectors on his clothes and bike by night. He should wear an approved helmet to protect his head.

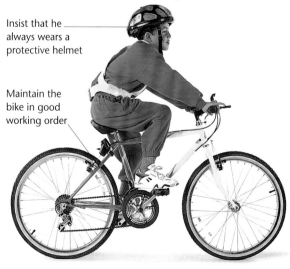

Insist that he always wears a protective helmet

Maintain the bike in good working order

## Where to play

What may seem common sense to you is not obvious to children.

- Show your child where it is safe to play – the playground, or local recreation ground, for example – and supervise him if necessary.
- Teach your child the dangers of playing in open areas, such as roads, building sites, and quarries.
- Tell your child not to play in the street, or on a pavement near the kerb – even if your street is quiet.
- Tell him that he must never chase a ball, a pet, or another child into the road.

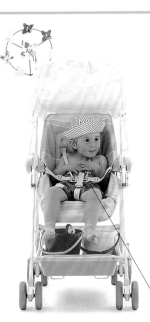

Harness your baby into his buggy

## Prams and buggies

- Never push a pram or buggy out into the traffic to see if the road is clear to cross. Pull the buggy to one side and check whether the road is safe. Remember that a child's buggy sticks out in front of you by at least 1m (3ft).
- When you park a pram or buggy, put on the brakes and point it away from traffic.
- Never tie your dog to the pram.
- Never leave a baby unattended.
- Keep your child away from the buggy when you are assembling or folding it to keep little fingers from being trapped.

## In the playground

All playgrounds should comply with safety standards; report any faulty equipment in community playgrounds to your local authority.

- The play area must be safely fenced off and away from roads.
- There should be a soft, even surface, such as bark chippings or rubber tiles, around equipment.
- Slides should be no higher than 2.4m (8ft) and preferably constructed on an earth mound to break any falls.
- Roundabouts should be low, with a smooth surface, designed so that young children can't get their feet stuck underneath.
- Climbing frames should be no higher than 2.4m (8ft), completely stable, and built over sand or a very soft surface to break falls.
- Swings for young children must have safety guards.
- There should be a clearly defined play area for toddlers and young children, set away from the more boisterous activities of older children.
- There should be someone to contact if any of the equipment is faulty.
- Dogs must not be allowed inside playgrounds.

Check that swings are set apart from main play equipment

> ## ⚠ IMPORTANT
>
> - **Remind** your child of the dangers of talking to strangers. Have a code word that a friend can use if colllecting your child. Tell your child not to go with anybody unless they use the code.

# Travelling with babies and children

Away from your home all the same rules of safety apply. However, you should be aware that the place you are staying in would not necessarily have been planned with young children in mind.

- If there is a swimming pool, never leave your child unattended in or near the water and, if there is a fence around it, keep the gate shut.
- Take baby milk and/or food with you as your child may not like what is available locally.

## Travelling abroad

- Make sure your child's immunisations are up to date. Some countries recommend additional vaccination, or anti-malaria medication; ask when booking a trip.
- Don't forget to take the necessary paperwork; babies and children need their own passports for most countries. It is a good idea to keep a photocopy of each passport (yours as well) in a separate bag.
- If you are hiring a car, always ask for child safety seats, or take your child's car seat with you.
- Make sure hire cars are fitted with sufficient safety belts and check that they are in good condition (not frayed) and working properly.
- Take insect repellent suitable for babies and young children, as they are particularly susceptible to insect bites. Apply the repellant in the early evening and again at bedtime when the insects are most active.
- Wash vegetables, salads, and fruit in cooled, boiled water or bottled water if there is any doubt about the local water.
- Boil water used to make up baby foods or milk.

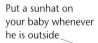

Put a sunhat on your baby whenever he is outside

## Air travel

- If booking tickets for children under the age of two, ask for seats where you can use a child safety seat or a sky cot.
- Give your baby a breastfeed, bottlefeed, or a dummy to suck as the plane ascends and descends because the change in pressure can cause earache in babies and children. Give an older child a sweet to suck, but make sure he does not choke on it.
- Take any food or milk that a baby needs on the journey. Airlines don't generally carry baby food, though they can often heat food or milk for you.
- Give your baby or child plenty to drink during the flight, to prevent dehydration.

## Sun protection

- Use sun block that protects your child from ultra violet A rays (UVA) and ultra violet B rays (UVB). The sun protector factor (SPF) numbers relate to UVA – chose SPF 30 – and a star-rating system indicates UVB protection. Re-apply regularly, especially after he has been in water. Use a cream that you know your child is not allergic to.
- Keep your baby or child's arms and legs covered as much as possible. Dress him in clothes made of closely woven fabric made of natural fibres.
- Make sure your child is protected by the shade in the middle of the day (about 10am until 4pm).
- Put a wide-brimmed hat on your child's head that covers his neck and face and use a parasol on a buggy.
- Give your child plenty to drink to prevent dehydration. If you are breastfeeding offer your baby more feeds; give a bottlefed baby plain water.

# Index

## A

## B

## C

# Acknowledgments

The publisher would like to thank the following for their kind permission to reproduce their photographs:
(Key: a-above; b-below/bottom; c-centre; f-far; l-left; r-right; t-top)
Jacket images: Front: Alamy Images: CJG - Lifestyle fclb; Getty Images: Tetra Images crb
All other images © Dorling Kindersley
For further information see: www.dkimages.com
Dorling Kindersley would like to thank:
Joe Mulligan, Head of First Aid Education, Nadine Threader, Jane Keogh, and Andrew Farrar from the British Red Cross; Cardiac Science for the loan of the paediatric AED; Hilary Bird for the index; the following for modelling:
**Children** Aleena Awan, Navaz Awan, Max Buckingham, Madeline Cameron, Alfie Clarke, Amy Davies, Thomas Davies, James Dow, Kyla Edwards, Austin Enil, Lia Foa, Maya Foa, Jessica Forge, Kashi Gorton, Emily Gorton, Thomas Greene, Alexander Harrison, Rupert Harrison, Ben Harrison, Jessica Harris-Voss, Hannah Headam, Jake Hutton, Rosemary Kaloki, Winnie Kaloki, Ella Kaye, Maddy Kaye, Jade Lamb, Emily Leney, Harriet Lord, Daniel Lord, Crispin Lord, Ailsa McCaughrean, Fiona Maine, Tom Maine, Kincaid Malik-White, Maija Marsh, Oliver Metcalf, Eloise Morgan, Tom Razazan, Jimmy Razazan, Georgia Ritter, Rebecca Sharples, Ben Sharples, Thomas Sharples, Ben Walker, Robyn Walker, Amy Beth Walton Evans, Hanna Warren-Green, Simon Weekes, Joseph Weir, Lily Ziegler.
**Adults** Shaila Awan, Claire le Bas, Joanna Benwell, Angela Cameron, Georgina Davies, Marion Davies, Sophie Dow, Tina Edwards, Rachel Fitchett, Emma Foa, Emma Forge, Caroline Greene, Susan Harrison, Victoria Harrison, Julia Harris-Voss, Roy Headam, Emma Hutton, Helga Lien Evans, Sylvie Jordan, Jane Kaloki, David Kaye, Louise Kaye, Philip Lord, Geraldine McCaughrean, Diana Maine, Brian Marsh, Jonathan Metcalf, Francoise Morgan, Juliette Norsworthy, Anna Pizzi, Hossein Razazan, Angela Sharples, John Sharples, Nadine Threader, Miranda Tunbridge, Vanessa Walker, Catherine Warren-Green, Toni Weekes, Robert Ziegler.
**Make-up:** Wendy Holmes, Pebbles, Geoff Portas.
**Additional photography** Andy Crawford, Steve Gorton, Ray Mollers, Suzannah Price, Dave Rudkin, Steve Shott, Lloyd Sturdy.

# Useful telephone numbers

IN AN EMERGENCY DIAL 999. ASK FOR THE AMBULANCE (medical emergencies only), FIRE BRIGADE, OR POLICE

FOR MEDICAL ADVICE CALL NHS DIRECT TELEPHONE 0845 4647

## Doctor
Name: _____
Address: _____
Telephone: _____
Out of hours telephone: _____
Surgery Hours: _____

## Health Visitor
Name: _____
Clinic Address: _____
_____
Telephone: _____
Clinic Hours: _____

## Dentist
Name: _____
Address: _____
Telephone: _____
Out of hours telephone: _____
Surgery Hours: _____

## Hospital Accident & Emergency
Address: _____
_____
Telephone: _____

## Late Night Chemist
Address: _____
Telephone: _____

## Local Police
Telephone: _____

## Gas Emergency Service
Telephone: _____

## Electricity Emergency Service
Telephone: _____

## Water Emergency Service
Telephone: _____

## British Red Cross

The British Red Cross runs first aid courses for all ages. For further information, get in touch with your local British Red Cross office; you will find the number in the telephone directory or in the Yellow Pages. Alternatively, visit www.redcross.org.uk/firstaid.

British Red Cross, UK Office
44 Moorfields, London, EC2Y 9AL

The Red Cross emblem is a symbol of protection during armed conflicts, and its use is restricted by law.

Details of the royalties payable to the British Red Cross can be obtained by writing to the publisher Dorling Kindersley at the following address:
80 Strand
London
WC2R 0RL